The Space Between

Cultivating Mindfulness, Peace, and Empowerment
In Your Life Through

Meta-Awareness, Framing, And Yoga

Andrew Paul Williams, Ph.D., E-RYT 500

Williams Press, LLC
Orange Park, Florida

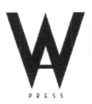

D1563932

Published in the United States by Williams Press, LLC,
Orange Park, Florida

Library of Congress Control Number: 2018912077

ISBN: 979-8361216055

The Space Between : Cultivating Mindfulness, Peace, and
Empowerment In Your Life Through Meta-Awareness,
Framing, And Yoga / Andrew Paul Williams

First U.S. Edition

The benefits I have experienced may be different from what you experience from these practices. I believe that if practiced regularly, Meta-Awareness, Framing, and Yoga can greatly improve the quality of anyone's life in terms of feeling more mindful, peaceful, and empowered, but these practices are not substitutes for professional care or medication. My suggestion to you in to use this educational information in addition to other resources, professional, and medical help as needed, and find whatever works best to meet your needs as you add these practices to your life to enhance what is going well and to help you in the areas you seek to improve.

For my mother,
LOIS VIRGINIA STRICKLAND WILLIAMS
who greatly encouraged me in my education, my Yoga
Teacher Training,
and as a Yoga instructor and worked with me to make this
book possible.
I love you and am grateful for all you have done to help me
with all my endeavors.

In memory of my father,
REVEREND GRADY H. WILLIAMS, SR.
who greatly encouraged me to pursue my education and
entrepreneurial endeavors.
Though he has been gone for many years, I have felt his
presence during this project
and through the good and challenging times. I think he would
be proud of this work.

Contents

Preface

This book grew out of my advanced 300-hour Yoga teacher training at Yoga Den in Jacksonville, Florida and the personal need to create space between being triggered by internal and external stimuli and responding—and especially working to become more responsive instead of reactive. The idea of writing about creating space between stimuli and my thoughts, emotions, body, and behaviors came to me after a practice led by Yoga Den Director, Alyson Foreacre about five years ago. Alyson mentioned creating space between our thoughts and our reactions as a benefit of Yoga at the closing of a special class, "Turkey Day Detox" she leads annually on Thanksgiving morning as a charitable fundraiser. This idea of creating space resonated with me and inspired me as I continued my 200 and 300 Hour Yoga Teacher Training, and this concept of creating space between thoughts and reactions became a large part of my personal practice and teaching over the past four years. As I worked with this idea that Alyson introduced us to, it evolved to for me as: Yoga creates space between stimuli and our thoughts, emotions, bodies, and behaviors—choosing with intent, responding instead of reacting, and this has become a mantra and guiding intention for me.

I was led to Yoga during my recovery from trauma, long-term respiratory problems, and chronic back and neck pain. During this recovery period I also found that going to Framing Theory—something I had worked with a great deal as graduate student, a researcher and professor—became invaluable in rediscovering my strengths and helping others too.

I rediscovered the concept Meta-Awareness during this time and found this mindfulness practice very helpful in learning to slow down and relax—ultimately allowing me to get in better touch with my inner wisdom and ability to choose with intent instead of reacting to my own thoughts, bad memories, fears about the future, physical pain, opinions of others, and the uncertainty that I felt overwhelmed by during this recovery period. Yoga became an important practice that integrated these concepts and was lifesaving and life changing for me, and as I finish my first 1,000 hours of teaching Yoga, I find that Meta-Awareness and Framing continue to shape my personal practice and teaching.

My intention for this book is to help you use the practices of Meta-Awareness, Framing, and Yoga to create space between stimuli—internal or external distractions, obstacles, and triggers—and your thoughts, emotions, body, and behaviors, choosing with intent, responding instead of reacting—creating more mindfulness, peace, and empowerment in your life.

I practice Meta-Awareness, Framing, and Yoga daily, and go to these practices when I'm challenged. I hope that they help you as they help me.

Namaste,

Andrew

Introduction: The Space Between

"Do you have the patience to wait till your mud settles and the water is clear?"

Lao Tzu

"Between stimulus and response there is a space.
In that space is our power to choose our response.
In our response lies our growth and our freedom."

Viktor E. Frankl, Holocaust Survivor

The Space Between

The Space Between is a place of clarity where we can cultivate mindfulness, peace, and empowerment in our lives.

In this space—and through the practice of pausing—we become more responsive and proactive instead of reactive.

In this space we can merge our intellect with our emotions and remove unnecessary emotional overlays that cloud our thoughts or negatively influence our behaviors.

In this space we become clearer, objective observers and also more actively engage in our lives and our experiences in healthier and more balanced ways.

In this space we find, and can become, our best authentic selves as we learn to align our thoughts and behaviors with our intentions, values, and spiritual beliefs.

In this space of greater clarity, we see that we have choices—often more choices than we initially realize, which is one of the many reasons why pausing and creating space is so important.

Creating the Space Between Helps You Cultivate Mindfulness, Peace, and Empowerment

There are myriad stimuli that we are exposed to in any given day and, if we are not careful, we will be reacting to internal and external distractions, obstacles, and triggers on a regular basis. In a typical day most of us are exposed to numerous media messages (including televised news, advertising, social media posts, and political news), interactions with people, dealing with traffic, physical sensations and pains, and our own thoughts about the past, present, and future.

These internal and external stimuli can often be distractions, obstacles, and triggers that can cause us to be reactive in our thoughts and behaviors, and these reactions take us away from mindfulness, peace, and empowerment.

In the classic science experiment Pavlov's dog wanted to eat every time it heard a bell ring. It was conditioned to do that. The bell was a trigger for the dog's reaction. This trigger affected the dog in numerous ways including physical behaviors. We often react similarly to internal and external triggers.

There are many different types of triggers. For example, a letter from the IRS, being cut off in traffic or being tailgated by an aggressive and angry driver, physical pain in your body, seeing an ex's social media posts with the new love of their live, excessive texting, and work or school stress can throw any of us out of balance.

Most of us struggle in some way or another with reacting to internal or external obstacles, triggers, or distractions—like Pavlovian dogs—where a stimulus triggers a knee-jerk reaction.

Again, keep in mind that there are many stimuli that can take us away from mindfulness, peace, and empowerment. For example, think of someone who really pushes your buttons—perhaps a coworker, boss, family member, or perhaps a politician with whom you strongly disagree with their stances, behaviors, or ways of communicating. Also, certain minor and major circumstances or some situations such as extreme weather, the death or illness of a loved one, traffic jams, or getting stuck in an airport due to flight delays can throw off the best of most of us. Sometimes it is our own physical pain or illness, bad memories, or fears and insecurities that trigger us. Often seemingly innocuous things like the time of day, a season of the year, a holiday, an event, the weather, a sound, a smell, or an environment can trigger feelings that negatively affect our thoughts and behaviors.

We are often conditioned to react immediately, mindlessly, and fearfully when we are triggered in our thoughts and our behaviors, and these thoughts and behaviors are often not in our best interests or in the best interests of others around us.

We all have places we go—or ways that we react first—when we are triggered, and often these reactive thoughts are behaviors are very knee-jerk and not representative of our best selves. For example, some of us get impatient or angry, some get anxious or afraid, and others freeze up and become immobilized when faced with something that challenges us.

While there are certainly many triggers that cause us to react and act impulsively, we often have patterns and standard negative go-to ways of thinking and acting when we are triggered that we need to acknowledge and address.

Most of us can relate to doing or saying things in haste in these reactive moments that we regret later. We all have some type of triggers, and learning to identify stimuli that take you away from mindfulness, peace, and empowerment will help you make healthier choices in terms of pausing.

Becoming aware of your patterns—what thoughts and behaviors take you towards and away from mindfulness, peace, and empowerment—will help you make better choices in this space between stimuli and your responses. Training ourselves to pause and create space between stimuli and choosing a response—instead of a reaction to a given stimulus—takes some work. Practicing the pause is like developing any skill or building muscle.

Through the practices of Meta-Awareness, Framing, and Yoga we create space between triggers and our responses—choosing with intent, responding instead of reacting. It takes time and effort to train and retrain ourselves to respond and be more proactive and responsive instead of reactive.

Developing the practice of pausing takes time and practice, and learning how to create this space allows us to be more positive and healthier as we choose thoughts and behaviors that are in alignment with our intentions, values, and spiritual beliefs. The numerous positive results in our lives worth the effort.

As we align our thoughts and our behaviors with our intentions, values and spiritual beliefs, we experience positive results internally and externally, and see many benefits in our lives:

As we practice pausing and creating the space between, we cultivate more mindfulness—slowing down, relaxing, and being more aware in the present moment—and become more thoughtful of ourselves, others, and the world around us;

As we practice pausing and creating the space between, we cultivate more peace—calmness and serenity—and become more relaxed and at ease with ourselves, others, and the world around us;

As we practice pausing and creating the space between, we cultivate more empowerment—confidence and healthy self-esteem—and become more comfortable, compassionate, efficacious, and empathetic, positive, and kind with our relationships with ourselves, others, and the world around us;

Our level of awareness itself increases as we learn to trust our inner wisdom and intuition more. We become clearer and more objective in assessing ourselves, others, and the world around us;

Our thoughts become clearer, more positive, and productive as we create space. We experience less cognitive dissonance, and we learn how to train and discipline our minds;

Our emotions become more balanced, calmer, and manageable as we gain a sense of efficacy and improved confidence in our ability to effectively manage internal and external triggers;

Our behaviors are improved by this level of clarity and we can improve on and increase behaviors that take us towards mindfulness, peace, and empowerment. We are also better able to check ourselves and stop or limit behaviors that have been problematic. We are better able to break cycles of spiraling in negative directions;

Our bodies and physical health benefit from making better choices driven by clarity and a greater mind body connection;

Our relationships with ourselves, others and the world around us are improved as we embrace reality and make healthier choices. There is a cyclical effect here because as we have a healthier relationship with ourselves, we improve our ability to positively relate with others and manage our lives in the world much more too, and of course, improved interactions help us feel better about ourselves; and

Our overall sense of congruence and improved alignment in all these parts of ourselves and our life experiences help us to feel more balanced and grounded—even when we are triggered or face major challenges. We live more with intent.

Practicing Creating The Space Between

An important way to create this space is to practice pausing— working to slow down, be more intentional, and noticing that you have choices.

Practicing Meta-Awareness, Framing, and Yoga on a regular basis helps us learn to slow down, pause, and create space between stimuli and our responses—cultivating more, mindfulness, peace, and empowerment in our lives.

As we learn to pause more and be more intentional with our thoughts and our behaviors, we can also go to the practices of Meta-Awareness, Framing, and Yoga at any time when we are feeling challenged and reactive.

As you begin these practices, I suggest that you think about what led you to this book. Take a little bit of time to get clear on the following questions as you prepare to work with the practices of Meta-Awareness, Framing, and Yoga.

What are your intentions?

What are your values?

What are your spiritual beliefs?

What does mindfulness mean to you?

What is your idea of peace?

What does empowerment mean to you?

What internal or external stimuli are distractions, obstacles, or triggers cause you to be reactive in your thoughts and behaviors and take you away from mindfulness, peace, and empowerment?

How would you prefer to respond to these stimuli?

What would your life look and feel like if you were more mindful, peaceful, and empowered?

Use your answers to these questions to guide your work with the practices of Meta-Awareness, Framing, and Yoga that are detailed in this book.

One of the biggest things I hope you take away from this book is that you have many choices—often more choices than you initially realize—and the practices of Meta-Awareness, Framing, and Yoga will help you see the numerous options available to you, especially when you are triggered and help you to live more with intent.

Chapter One Meta-Awareness

"The man who is aware of himself is henceforward independent."

Virginia Woolf

"The key to growth is the introduction of higher dimensions of consciousness into our awareness."

Lao Tzu

Meta-Awareness

Meta-Awareness is simply the awareness of your awareness.

Meta-Awareness is a mindfulness practice where we make awareness itself the main point of concentration and focus. In other words, you essentially focus on your awareness and notice what you notice.

The fact that your mind is so incredible that you can be aware of your own awareness is an amazing thing—and a practical one too.

You have the ability to be the observer of your life, and through clearly observing comes the ability to transcend and move through minor or major internal or external triggers that challenge you.

You can use your awareness to create more mindfulness, peace, and empowerment in your life by letting your awareness itself become a filter through which you process what you are noticing internally and externally.
This noticing—without judgment—is a hallmark of mindfulness practice, and your ability to scan your life, to evaluate, and to make healthy choices in terms of your thoughts and behaviors helps you be more present and engaged in your life experiences—instead of feeling like life is just happening to you.

Through Meta-Awareness you mindfully engage with, process, and respond to reality—not avoiding it by just being the observer and watching yourself and experiences cinematically, like you're at an either good or bad movie—but by using the clarity you gain from observing to make better choices in your thoughts and behaviors.

Meta-Awareness is a practice of clarity and engagement—not distance and detachment. You can view this higher level of awareness as your inner wisdom, your higher self, the best you, or your intuition.

Meta-Awareness is essentially our higher level of thinking and processing, and we can use this improved, clearer thinking to choose healthier thoughts and behaviors. These are the two things in life we can really control: We can choose our thoughts, and we can choose our behaviors.

Through the practice of Meta-Awareness, we can mindfully step back and observe our thoughts, emotions, bodies, behaviors, and our awareness itself, and we develop an improved sense of clarity—even when we feel triggered.

This level of awareness is a huge accomplishment, but it is applying Meta-Awareness and using that level of clear mindfulness—to respond rather than react and merge our emotions with our intellect, to be both the clear observer and active participant in our lives— where we claim and create empowerment and peace.
This does not mean we eliminate or fix all our issues by just observing. What it does mean is that we gain clarity and are able to manage our issues, and internal or external challenges, by making healthier choices.

Even with this greater awareness, we all have many different internal and external stimuli that can distract, block, and trigger—throwing us off balance, making us more reactive than proactive or responsive. Through the clarity we achieve from the practice of Meta-Awareness, we can get in touch with our true and best selves.

Meta-Awareness Helps You Cultivate Mindfulness, Peace and Empowerment

First and foremost, by practicing Meta-Awareness we can mindfully choose thoughts and behaviors that are in alignment with our intentions, values, and spiritual beliefs, and through making these healthier choices we become more peaceful and empowered.

As we work to become more mindful—more aware of our thoughts, emotions, bodies, behaviors, others, the world around us, our triggers, and our options—we gain clarity and more healthy engagement with our life experiences. We are more able to build on our strengths and better manage our weaknesses. We become more thoughtful and considerate of ourselves and others.
We take this mental step back as an observer to gain a sense of objectivity and to get in touch with, accept, and address reality—not to avoid reality.

As we gain objectivity we can see how emotional overlays cloud our judgment and negatively affect our thoughts, emotions, and behaviors.
This clarity takes some work because many of us have developed maladaptive strategies for coping with things in life that emotionally trigger us, and our perspectives are often shaped more by feelings than facts.

We often have immediate, go-to emotionally-reactive thought and behavior patterns that we turn to on a sort of autopilot, and unfortunately, many of these go-to patterns of thoughts and behaviors can be harmful to ourselves and others in minor or major ways.

As we gain this awareness and notice our triggers, our patterns, and the consequences of our reactive choices—and if we can do so without judgment, but instead with compassion for ourselves, using discernment and our own inner wisdom to make responsive choices—we can break free of ways of reacting that rob us of the mindfulness, peace, and empowerment that we really want in our lives.

One way of looking at Meta-Awareness is that we become more empathetic with ourselves and develop a greater sense of efficacy in our ability to see ourselves and our patterns with clearer vision—and through acknowledging this ability to manage life from a greater place of awareness—we can make better decisions in terms of what we think and what we do.

The practice of Meta-Awareness helps us to be more present and actualized people—not getting bogged down in a victim mode or beating ourselves up. The victim persona (or archetype) is as narcissistic as the braggart, and the vicious cycle of judging ourselves, staying depressed and anxious, and focusing on our faults or negative storyline does not lead us toward mindfulness, peace, or empowerment.

Seeing ourselves clearly—and using this clarity to make adjustments in our thoughts and behaviors—does help to free us from being stuck in some sort of negative, reactive, and mindless loop, and while it sounds simple, this process of gaining clarity and improving our thoughts and behaviors takes time and practice.

The intention and the benefit of Meta-Awareness is gaining a healthy sense of self and a balanced perspective. From this healthier perspective, we can make better choices that improve all aspects of our lives.

Again, it is both through noticing on purpose—and mindfully choosing to align our thoughts and behaviors with our intentions, values, and spiritual beliefs—that we find the benefits of this practice, and the benefits are numerous.

Practicing Meta-Awareness

Practicing Meta-Awareness is a straightforward process of taking a mental step back and being the observer of your own awareness and all areas of your life—noticing without judgement and acknowledging your own inner wisdom.

This is a process of gaining clarity, objectivity, getting in touch with reality, and being more present for your experiences.

It is through the recognition of your choices—and then using this recognition to make healthy decisions about how you think and behave—that you become more mindful, peaceful, and empowered

Start this practice with slowing down, taking a mental step back, and become aware of what you notice.

Let your awareness itself be the starting point for this mindfulness practice.

The fact that you are able to be aware of the fact that you are aware is a significant accomplishment. Please just take a moment and think about how important gaining this ability really is and the positive impact it can have on your life.

This level of awareness leads to greater clarity, and it is perhaps the highest level of awareness. Take time to notice and observe yourself on multiple levels.

Get comfortable with the idea of being the observer.

In his groundbreaking book, *The Untethered Soul*, Michael Singer suggests that the real us is the one that notices our thoughts, emotions, behaviors, bodies, and so forth. I agree and like the idea that the real us can step back from our own thoughts, emotions, and behaviors in order to observe and choose.

Notice what you notice.

This is the crux of the practice of Meta-Awareness. Focus on your awareness—this higher level of thinking, your intuition, or whatever you want to call this place of clarity. You can think of it as your internal friend, higher wisdom, the God within you, or perhaps even as an angel that is looking out for you on one shoulder telling you not to break your diet, not to send the angry e-mail when you are upset, or not to give in to an addictive pattern. The simple idea is that you have a greater awareness that you can get in touch with if you take a mental and emotional step back, relax, and allow yourself to notice what you notice.

Focus on your awareness and the ability to check in with yourself. You can just slow down and take a few minutes to notice what you are aware of. It doesn't have to take long to do this, but it does take practice. In many ways this process just seems like common sense and discipline, but we all have different things we struggle with in terms of our thoughts, emotions, and behaviors. We all can benefit from this focus on our awareness and gaining clarity because we can use this practice to become our own wise counselor, friend, parent, or teacher who has our own best interest at heart. Through Meta-Awareness we take better care of ourselves. This is a practical and powerful skill.

From this point of clarity—and focusing on your awareness itself—use this place of objectivity to look at yourself and your life. Really step back and notice your:

Awareness;

Thoughts;

Emotions and Mental Health;

Body and Physical Health;

Behaviors;

Relationship with Self, Others, and The World Around You;

Management of Resources (for example, Time, Energy, Money);

Intentions;

Values;

Spirituality and Spiritual beliefs;

Fears and Insecurities;

Distractions, Obstacles, and Triggers;

Reactions (that is, emotionally reactive thoughts and behaviors that take you away from being mindful, peaceful, and empowered);

Responses (that is, responsive thoughts and behaviors that merge your intellect with your emotions and help you stay mindful, peaceful, and empowered); and

Choices, the energy behind your choices, and the outcomes of your choices.

Evaluate what you notice in all of these areas in your life. As the objective observer, assess your life in large and small ways, and see what is taking your either toward or away from being mindful, peaceful, and empowered.

From these observations and greater awareness, be honest with yourself about what is working well and what isn't. Don't be a harsh critic. Be clear but not critical as you see things that need minor or major improvement. Remove any unnecessary emotional overlays you may have, and just be honest with yourself about your strengths and weaknesses in these areas.

It can be very difficult to step back and just be an accurate observer with ourselves—especially when it comes to parts of our lives that we struggle with, but this honest assessment will help you make better choices.

We often go to great lengths to avoid facing difficult realties because it is quite painful to face the shadow aspects of ourselves and our lives. This tough look in the mirror can be especially hard because we often lie to ourselves and tell stories to reinforce beliefs and roles that we have grown accustomed to. But paradoxically it is through humbly admitting our character flaws and weaknesses that we gain the strength to address them with dignity and resolve.

Taking an honest evaluation of yourself can guide you to better choices in terms of your thoughts and behaviors in these areas of your life that you have assessed.

Make mindful choices based on these assessments, and make adjustments as needed to your thoughts and your behaviors that are in alignment with your intentions, values, and spiritual beliefs.

Start with small steps as you work to make more mindful choices and do a little along. For example, if you come to realize that you think too much or too little about yourself, start coming up with ways to become more balanced in your thinking.

The same goes for if you are harsh in your assessment of others—or if you are in a habit of putting people on pedestals and then being disappointed. It will take time to shift your thinking about yourself and others to a more neutral place if you have tended to skew either very positive or negative.

By being honest with yourself about your inflated or deflated perceptions of yourself or others, you can be more honest as you move forward and learn from your patterns.

Take some time to especially focus on gaining clarity and improving your thoughts and your behaviors. Don't try to over adjust. Often just minor improvements in our choices get us remarkable results.

Try building on what you feel are your strengths and addressing your weaknesses. For example, if you know that you overeat a lot because of depression or anxiety, a crash diet is probably not going to really help you find peace and empowerment. A quick fix doesn't really become sustainable or create lasting change.

Look at what thoughts and emotions are leading you to overeating (or spending, drinking, yelling, etc.).

When you start to eat too much or whatever an excessive activity may be for you, ask yourself why you are doing this and what thoughts or emotions are driving this behavior.
Then address the behavior in a few different ways. First, try to make little modifications to the behavior itself and come up with a few things you can do that are healthier when you are triggered. Second, think about how you can shift your thoughts to minimize whatever emotion is affecting you and leading to the actions that are taking you out of balance and out of alignment with your intentions, values, and spiritual beliefs.

This process of becoming mindful and then choosing better thoughts and behaviors is an ongoing one—especially for any of us who have developed maladaptive coping habits. But it is an ongoing process guided by awareness that will lead to better choices on a daily basis and help you create new habits that create more mindfulness, peace, and empowerment in your life.

As you continue to regularly scan your life, your thoughts, emotions, body, behaviors, and relationships, come up with ways to think and behave that you feel are improvements and keep doing that.

If you have harmful thought or behavioral patterns, you will need to let your awareness of these guide you to creating strategies and tactics to help keep yourself in alignment with your intentions, values, and spiritual beliefs that take you more towards mindfulness, peacefulness, and empowerment.

You can do this by making time for checking in and creating a structure that supports you in making better choices—and helps prevent you from continuing to make harmful ones.

Get clear about what your strengths are.

Get clear about what your challenges are.

Get clear what led you to this book.

Be honest about what thoughts and behaviors are helping or hurting you. Come up with ways to choose better. If you need professional support in doing this work and making improvements, get it.

Overcoming your challenges will become easier when you focus on awareness and choose to improve your thoughts and behaviors as a way of daily life.

Repeat the process of noticing, evaluating, and choosing.

This is an ongoing, cyclical process—not a linear one with a starting point and a finish line. Developing a regular Meta-Awareness practice will yield positive results in your life.

Make Meta-Awareness a daily practice—perhaps developing short morning, afternoon, and evening routines—and using weekly, monthly, and yearly dedicated times to practice this noticing of what you notice and evaluating how it is helping you. Find what works best for you, and keep doing this practice.

Going To Meta-Awareness When You Feel Challenged

In addition to practicing Meta-Awareness on a regular basis, this practice is something you can draw on in times when you feel triggered in any way.

If you are feeling triggered by any internal or external stimuli that is a distraction or obstacle in your life, use this process of noticing, evaluating, and choosing thoughts and behaviors that support your intentions, values, and spiritual beliefs to skillfully manage your way through and help you become more mindful, peaceful, and empowered.

You can always go to the practice of Meta-Awareness.

Chapter Two: Framing

"The mind is its own place
and in itself, can make a Heaven of Hell, a Hell of Heaven."

John Milton

"The greatest discovery of any generation is that
a human being can alter his life by altering his attitude."

William James

Framing

Framing is the process of how we interpret reality and all the stimuli to which we are exposed. Framing is not just what we focus on, but more importantly, Framing is how we process and perceive information to which we are exposed.

Often, how we see things is as important—or even more important—than what is actually happening. This is true in a very large sense, in terms of our overall worldview and in smaller ways, in terms of our daily life experiences.

For example, if we choose to view something as a problem our experience will be guided by that perception of dealing with a problem. If we see something just as a situation, we have a more neutral and matter-of-fact response to it. If we see something as an opportunity, our experience will be guided by finding ways to make the most of it.

Our perception shapes our reality and affects our thoughts, emotions, and behaviors to a large degree, and we have the ability to choose our perspective.

Like it sounds, Framing is a process of putting things in a frame—essentially a frame of reference in your mind.

Think of using Instagram—or how you take and edit a photo using any camera, program, or app. You focus, you choose what you want to focus on, perhaps cropping later, and then you may do some editing in terms of brightness, and so on. You can similarly do the same thing with how you view yourself, others, issues, objects, situations, and events.

Think of these adjustments to your thinking like editing or using a filter on a camera or Instagram. Often little adjustments to a photo change and improve not only that focus, but also the quality, clarity, and the mood/feel of the picture too. Refocusing and adjusting your Framing has this effect on your perception of life too.

Whether it is a large world view or just a tendency to be more positive or negative, our Framing shapes our lives in large and small ways—bigtime and in realtime. What we focus on—and how we focus—affects our thoughts, emotions, bodies and physical health, behaviors, and relationships with ourselves, others, and the world around us.

Framing Helps You Cultivate Mindfulness, Peace, and Empowerment.

Framing is essentially how we organize reality and process our life experiences. It is a very powerful practice. We often do this on a sort of autopilot.

By examining your Framing patterns—and making conscious choices to Frame or Reframe—you can gain many positive results in your life.

There are myriad stimuli that we are exposed to in a given day. From the time we wake up in the morning to the time we go to bed at night our senses are bombarded with information. Some of this information is helpful, some is hurtful, some is important, some is meaningless, some is funny, and some is sad.

If we are not very careful we could be pulled around mentally and emotionally by the flood of stimuli we are exposed to daily from the mass media, social media, people we encounter at work and in school, emails, phone calls and texts, and our interpersonal communications. Our senses are literally bombarded daily, and the number of stimuli that we are exposed to in a on a regular basis is staggering. There is a lot to process—both internal and external.

We must set boundaries with others, and we must also learn to filter ourselves in terms of what we think, say, and do if we want to become mindful, peaceful, and empowered. If we do not choose wisely what we focus on, how much time and energy we use focusing, and the ways we focus, we will be reacting to external and internal stimuli all the time.

Many of us practice Framing without realizing that we have choices. But make no mistake about it, Framing is a choice.

We can be proactive and intentional and set our focus, we can be responsive and merge our intelligence with our emotions as we process life, or we can emotionally react to stimuli and have our thoughts and behaviors dictated by external or internal distractions and obstacles to mindfulness, peace, and empowerment.

As you learn to notice your Framing patterns, you can develop an understanding of what the energy is behind what you focus on and how you focus—and what the results of your Framing processes are. Based on the outcomes you see, you can then reinforce what is working well for you—or refocus as needed to better align your Framing with your intentions, values, and spiritual beliefs.

Through the practice of Framing, we are able to become more intentional in our thought process—in terms of what we choose to focus on, how much time and energy we spend on what we focus on, and how we choose to perceive what we focus on.

These mindful Framing choices can take us towards more mindfulness, peace, and empowerment. Framing can become deliberate act of shaping your own reality—a reality that is in alignment with your intentions, values, and spiritual beliefs.

Practicing Framing

Through the practice of Framing we can intentionally shape how we think and feel about our life and life experiences—people, issues, events, places, the past, the present, the future, and ourselves.

We can achieve positive results from Framing by being mindful in choosing what we focus on, how much time and energy we use on what we focus on, the ways we focus, and shifting our perspectives and readjusting our focus and Reframing how we look at things as needed.

Think about what you focus on how and much time and energy you use focusing.

Choosing with intent what we focus on and how much time and energy we spend focusing can serve us greatly in helping us to cultivate mindfulness, peace, and eempowerment in our lives. What you focus on will shape your reality.

What are you focusing on from the time you wake up in the morning until you go to bed at night?

When you wake up in the morning are you spending some time focused on things that take you towards or away from mindfulness, peace, and empowerment? Are you priming yourself to see the best or worst in yourself, others, and the world around you as you start you day?

Who is setting your frames for you? Are you choosing what you focus on, how much you focus, the ways you focus, or are others choosing this for you? Who is setting your agenda—in terms of what you think about and how you think about those things?

Do you focus more on what is right or wrong with yourself, others, and the world around you?

What amount of time and energy to you spend on media (including social media, phone, computer, and tablet) usage?

Are you more focused on the past, present or the future?
Are you focused more on your own fearfulness or on your hopes and dreams?

Are you Framing things in ways that support and motivate you towards your intentions?

Are you Framing things in ways that are congruent with what is important to you and congruent with your values?

Are you Framing things in ways that are congruent with your spiritual beliefs?

Think about the ways you focus and Frame your life and life experiences.

Take time to evaluate how you think and talk about anything to others and to yourself.

Your words matter a lot. Look at the adjectives you use to describe issues, events, people, places, things, and especially yourself and your life experiences.

What is the tone of your dialogue? Is it positive, negative, or neutral?

Are you having compassion for yourself and others in your descriptions, or are you being critical and judgmental? Of course, we all need to evaluate and discern to make good choices. But are you overly critical and harsh in your perspective?

Are you being substantive or ambiguous in how you describe things? Often vague descriptions can be powerful and more of a positive or negative emotional cue, and specific language can better help merge your intelligence more with your emotions. Get clear on your words choices about how you describe anything to improve clarity of your thoughts and emotions—and positively influence your behaviors.

Are you focusing on what's right, or what's wrong? Are you going to gratitude—even if something is challenging? A focus on gratitude can have a huge impact in improving your thoughts, feelings, and behaviors. As you look at how you describe things, are you coming from a place of gratitude, or are you taking things for granted or perhaps focused on what is wrong or lacking? If you are coming from a place of scarcity, you will focus more on what is called a poverty consciousness. If you are focused on how much is good or right, you will have more thoughts and feelings of abundance. These thoughts and feelings will influence your behaviors and shape your reality—thus become a sort of self-fulfilling prophecy.

Using humor can be a real game changer in shifting your thoughts, emotions, and behaviors—especially if you can laugh at yourself and your own experiences. Laughter can be very healing and therapeutic. As you look at how you describe things and how you evaluate minor or major things in your life on a given day, do you have a sense of humor at all, or are you taking everything very seriously? If you are uptight, you'll probably notice more tension in your body and negative emotions. If you can laugh some and have a humorous perspective especially about yourself, you'll probably feel more relaxed physically and have more positive emotions—even when things may be far from perfect. Framing with humor can benefit you a great deal on all levels of your life.

Use affirmations and positive statements that are in alignment with your intentions, values, and spiritual beliefs as ways to help you shape and reinforce mindful, peaceful and empowering perspectives about yourself, your life, your experiences, others, and the world around you.

Notice what metaphors you use to describe things. Is life a journey or a struggle? How do you describe yourself and your life experiences?

Find quotes, verses, sayings, perhaps something from a book or short story, a TV show, movie, or even lyrics from a song that you like to call to mind and help you have something to focus on and to shift your perspective when needed.

Consider using a mantra—something that you can repeat and go to on a regular basis to calm your mind and help you Frame minor and major things in ways that are congruent with your intentions, values, and spiritual beliefs.

Notice your storyline. What is your story? Is it a tragedy or a comedy? What stories are you telling yourself about your life and your life experiences. Take time to identify what stories you are telling about yourself your life, other, and the world around you— about life itself. We all create narratives to understand our lives and process reality. How is your story working for you?

What role or roles are you playing in your life—personally and professionally? Are you the hero or the victim in your story? How do you view and describe yourself? Understanding your archetypes and archetypal patters can help you understand your thoughts, emotions, and behaviors.

Notice what is taking you away from feeling and acting mindful, peaceful, and empowered.

Consider your choices in terms of what you are focusing on, how much energy or time you are expending, and the ways you are Framing an issue, situation, person, or yourself.

Notice ways your Framing choices are in—or out of—alignment with your intentions, values, and spiritual beliefs.

Reinforce what is in alignment, and Reframe what is not.

You have many choices with Framing and Reframing that will help you improve your life on all levels.

Use Reframing when needed to shift your perspective to one that takes you towards mindfulness, peace and empowerment—and is in alignment with your intentions, values, and spiritual beliefs.

How is the way you view things working for you?

What do your thoughts, feelings, body, behaviors, and relationships tell you about the outcome of how you frame things?

If you feel out of balance or frustrated in any area, there is a good chance that you will benefit greatly from learning to Reframe what you are focusing on and perhaps shift your focus.

Reframing is a powerful technique. Often a minor shift in Framing will produce large positive results. Learn to identify the ways in which your Framing is helping or hurting you. Build on what is working well and use Reframing to improve what is not serving you.

For example, you can change just one word. Perhaps you notice a difference in describing yourself as working through something instead of saying that you are having a tough time.

Notice what is going on in terms of Framing in your life, evaluate, and adjust what you're focusing on, how much energy you're using, how you are focusing, or how you are focusing by Reframing if needed.

Using Framing and Reframing When You Feel Challenged

Being intentional with your Framing on a regular basis will help you improve your life in many areas, and it is a practice that can easily become a part of your daily life.

If you notice yourself feeling triggered, take a step back and think about the choices you are making regarding what you are focusing one, the amount of time and energy you are using to focus, the ways that you are focusing.

You can always go to this practice of Framing with intent—and Reframing as needed—when you notice that you feel challenged by internal or external distractions, obstacles, and triggers.

Chapter Three: Yoga

"Yoga is the settling of the mind into silence. When the mind has settled, we are established in our essential nature, which is unbounded Consciousness. Our essential nature is usually overshadowed by the activity of the mind."

Patanjali

"Yoga is the journey of the self, through the self, to the self."

The Bhagavad Gita

Yoga

Yoga is an eight-part practice—a set of guidelines and exercises—that includes ethical restraints, lifestyle observances, breathwork, postures and movements, and mind training.

Yoga is much more than just a physical practice.

If you practice any of the eight limbs of Yoga, you are practicing Yoga.

Yoga helps us cultivate balance—mentally, physically, and spiritually.

Yoga can be practiced by anyone, at any place, and at any time.

There is not just one way to practice Yoga. There are many great traditions and approaches to the practice Yoga for you to choose from as you find what is right for you—as you develop a personal and sustainable Yoga practice.

There are many ways to practice Yoga—in the studio/on the mat and in the world—throughout our daily lives.

Yoga is much simpler and more straightforward than it is often presented.

If you can breathe, you can practice Yoga.

The Eight Limbs of Yoga

Limb One: *Yamas – Integrity with Others and the World—Moral or Ethical Restraints*

Ahimisa: Nonviolence/Nonharming and Kindness
Satya: Truthfulness
Asteya: Nonstealing
Brahmacharya: Moderation and Self-Control/Management
Aparigraha: Non-Hoarding /Non-Greed/Grasping, Generosity

Limb Two: Niyamas *– Integrity with Yourself—Lifestyle Observances*

Saucha: Purity and Cleanliness
Santosha: Contentment and Gratitude
Tapas: Willpower and Discipline
Svadhyaya: Self-Study and Contemplation
Ishvara Pranidhana: Devotion/Commitment to Spiritual Growth and Development/ Self Study and Focus on Higher Good

Limb Three: *Asanas – The Physical Practice*

The physical practice of moving your body into shapes and postures. There are many types of Yoga postures that range from beginner to advanced. These include seated, standing, spine, prone, twists, back bends, inversions, balancing, and restorative shapes. These asanas can be adapted and modified for people who are in excellent physical condition and for people who are limited in their strength and mobility.

Limb Four: *Pranayama – Controlled Breathing*

There are numerous breath exercises that can be a part of a Yoga practice. Controlled, mindful, and deeper breathing are an important part of Yoga, and there are numerous breath exercises that benefit you in terms of your mental clarity, emotional balance, and physical energy level.

Limb Five: *Pratyahara – Sensory Withdrawal*

Training your mind to withdraw from the senses and go within is a significant part of the practice of Yoga. Allowing yourself to relax and let go of past and future, internal and external obstacles or distractions, worry or fear is a huge accomplishment and helps you get to a calm place in your mind.

Limb Six: *Dharana – Concentration and Focus*

Focusing the mind is another key part of the mental training in Yoga. Finding a point of focus helps you to quiet mental chatter and calm your active mind.

Limb Seven: *Dhyana – Meditation*

Learning to get to a calm mind—or experience stillness—takes a good bit of practice, and the ability to quiet your mind is often accomplished by going through the other limbs first.

Limb Eight: *Samadhi – Union or Bliss*

Getting to a place where you feel enlightened or connected is an intention of your Yoga practice. These moments are often fleeting, but when you feel grounded, content, and a sense of balance and harmony, you know it.

There are no shortcuts to finding *Samadhi*, but there are many ways you can practice the other seven limbs of Yoga to get you to this incredible state. Not to be confused with a sort of high—this is a genuine relaxed place of true mindfulness, peace, and empowerment that is unique and different for each person who practices Yoga.

Yoga Helps Cultivate Personal Power and Peace

Through the practice of Yoga, we can link philosophy—ethical restraints and lifestyle observances—with physical shapes and movements, controlled breathing, and mind control and meditation to create balance in our lives and become more mindful, peaceful, and empowered.

Yoga helps us be more flexible and develop strength in our minds and in our bodies. Yoga creates space in our bodies and in our minds. Yoga helps us mentally, physically and spiritually.

Yoga is not a religion, but it can certainly help a person of spiritual beliefs to deepen their religious practices through practicing intention setting and prayer as a part of the Yoga practice, which can also include using verses or sacred texts as a mantra. Someone who is not religious may develop a deeper connection with the universe, the world around them, nature, science, others, and themselves that is more energetic and metaphysical than they have experienced before practicing Yoga.

The practice of Yoga is transformative for the person who participates in any of the many physical or mental exercises or who follows the instructions relating to themselves and others through a structured or informal practice.

Yoga helps us be more accepting of ourselves, others, and the world around us. It helps us develop a kinder and more compassionate perspective that is shaped by seeing others, ourselves and the world around us with clearer vision, kind eyes, and compassion.

This kind and realistic perspective helps us make peace with reality and what is—instead of trying to impose our personal judgments and biases of what things should be. This acceptance and clarity that we gain through Yoga helps us become more peaceful and empowered in our lives as we learn to go with the flow instead of resisting it.

Practicing Yoga

Taking the time to have a dedicated practice that incorporates all eight limbs is a very rewarding experience. It is always an option to practice some parts of Yoga as we go through our daily lives. You can view your Yoga practice as something you do on the mat or in the world, and I encourage you to do both.

Making dedicated time for a structured practice yields many benefits, and there is something remarkable about experiencing the shared energy while practicing with a group in a studio. Blocking out time to a personal practice at home is also very rewarding. You will also find that you can go to any aspect of Yoga that resonates with you to help you when you are challenged.

Taking time to literally roll out your mat (or sit in a chair) and practice Yoga is a wonderful thing that allows you to benefit from all eight limbs. You can also find ways to focus on each limb during dedicated practice, and you will also find that you can practice Yoga off the mat in your daily life.

Below you will find suggestions for each limb, as well as an integrated Eight-Limb practice. Suggestions for dedicated practice (on the mat) and in your daily life (off the mat) are detailed too.

Here are some ways to practice the eight limbs of Yoga individually and together as a more structured practice. Taking the time to get familiar with each of the eight limbs will help you find opportunities to enrich your life and ways to respond to distractions, obstacles, and triggers.

Developing a regular practice that incorporates all the limbs is beneficial on many levels. Examples of how to practice the eight limbs of Yoga are provided below, and a sample integrated practice that is like the ones I teach in the studio is included at the end of this book.

An Important Note Regarding Safety, Benefits, and Contraindications:

There are many benefits to the breath and physical exercises in a Yoga practice. There are also numerous cautions. I've provided several the most commonly used exercises that I find helpful for myself and my students.

Before you do any of these, please take some time to research them, get professional instruction, use books or online materials to ensure that you are doing them safely.

Also, please consult your physician before doing these breath and physical exercises. If you have any medical conditions or have had surgery, you need to be especially cautious with starting your breath and physical practice. These two limbs of Yoga can help most people, and they can be modified to accommodate for disabilities.

It is important that you use caution and get professional guidance for these to avoid injury or exacerbating any current illness or condition.

Practicing Limb One: Yamas – Integrity with Others/the World— Moral/Ethical Restraints

Ashima – Nonviolence/Nonharming and Kindness

Ashima On the Mat: In terms of your personal practice, think of ways to be kind to yourself and honoring where you are, and not comparing yourself to anyone else or any other time in your life as you move through the shapes and never force anything that doesn't feel right for you. Also, take time to think about your wishes for other people and the world as a part of your practice. Are there people in your life you could be kinder to in terms of how you think about them, how you talk to them, or how you behave towards them? Are you doing what you can to make the world a better place? Think about ways you can treat others and the world around you just a little bit better, and make it your intention to do so.

Ashima In the World: Find opportunities to demonstrate your kind thoughts though your words and behaviors. Demonstrate compassion to others by looking for ways to lift up situations when you feel frustrated or disappointed. Sometimes saying nothing at all is the kindest thing to do if your words or behaviors would be hurtful to others.

Satya – Truthfulness

Satya On the Mat: In terms of your personal practice, be honest with yourself about your energy level and any pain or limitations you may be experiencing and don't overdo anything just because you see a teacher or another student doing something that doesn't feel right for you.
Also, take time to think about how truthful you are in your relationships with others and the world around you. Set the intention to be more honest with how you present yourself and in your personal and professional interactions. Think about ways where you feel you may have not been truthful and consider opportunities to correct and improve those areas.

Satya In the World: Try to be as honest, truthful, and transparent as possible and appropriate in your thoughts, words, and behaviors.

Asteya – Nonstealing

Asteya On the Mat: Think about ways in which you can make sure that you are not taking away from others in terms of their time, energy, money, or other resources, and make the commitment to be more Mindful in your interactions with others so you ensure that you are not taking what does not belong to you. Set the intention to behave in ways that reinforce the belief in yourself that you have enough and that you are enough.

Asteya In the World: Be cautious in your dealings to make sure that you are not taking what is not yours in any way. Be on time, be generous, and be respectful of other peoples' time energy, money, possessions, relationships, and other resources. Do your part, and act with confidence that you have all you need so that you do not act in any way that takes away from others. If you have an area in your life where you have been acting needy—or coming from a place of scarcity—be honest with yourself about having this poverty consciousness, own it, and improve the level of your thoughts and behaviors in this weak area. Make sure to give credit and acknowledge others.

Brahmacharya – Moderation and Self-Control/Management

Brahmacharya On the mat: Take time to think about your life and any way that you feel you are out of balance or excessive in your thoughts, words, or behaviors, and set the intention to be more moderate and balanced in these areas. Are there habits in your life—even things that are considered healthy and positive—that you have taken to extreme and lost balance? Perhaps there are some obstacles and distractions in disguise in your life?

Brahmacharya In the world: As you go through your daily life, be more intentional and mindful with your thoughts, words, and behaviors in terms of any excessive or addictive tendencies you may have. This can be in terms of eating, drinking, substances, shopping, gambling, exercise, work, sex, media usage, talking, or anything that you know can be compulsive or addictive for you in your life. Acknowledging these areas and working on them, with support if needed, can be a huge part of your Yoga practice.

Aparigraha – Nonhoarding/Nongreed/Nongrasping and Generosity

Aparigraha On the Mat: Take time to think about ways in your life that you may be grasping, hoarding, or greedy in any way and set the intention to let go of those behaviors and visualize ways that you can be more generous.

Aparigraha In the World: Find ways in your daily life to demonstrate generosity in your thoughts, words, and behaviors with others. Clean out your physical space at home or office and donate things you don't enjoy and use. Find ways to share your time, energy, and talent with others.

Practicing Limb Two: *Niyamas – Integrity with Yourself— Lifestyle Observances*

Saucha – Purity and Cleanliness.

Saucha On the Mat: Take some time to think about ways you can clean and purify your life. Work on letting go of and improving negative thoughts, harmful emotions, self-destructive behaviors, improving your diet, improving the way you take care of yourself, organizing your home, detailing your car, sorting out your office, and so forth. Think about areas you'd like to clean out and improve in your life and visualize how things will look and feel when you do so. Using your breath and movements as a metaphor for the idea of bringing in what is positive and eliminating what is harmful—and does not serve you—can help you integrate this important part of Yoga philosophy with your mental and physical practice.

Saucha In the World: Find ways in your daily life to clean and declutter in your home, office, care, yard, and so forth. Throw away unneeded things, recycling, donating, and giving them away to those who can enjoy them is one way to practice. Look at your schedule and free up activities that clutter your life. Evaluate your relationships and limit or eliminate those that are unhealthy or toxic for you. Clear your mind of negative and fearful thoughts. Improve the quality of your diet. Evaluate your media diet and social media usage as well as texting, emails, and phone calls to see if you can cut back some in these areas. Find opportunity to clean and purify your life.

Santosha – Contentment and Gratitude

Santosha On the Mat: Honor where you are by not comparing yourself with anyone else or any other time in your life. Focus on gratitude and appreciation and contentment in your life and for your Yoga practice.

Santosha In the World: Take time in the morning to start your day with a focus on gratitude and think about what you are thankful for through prayer or meditation. Throughout your day put an effort into slowing down, noticing, and appreciating your life, nature, other people, food, your home, work, and what you have in the present moment, and demonstrate your appreciation through your words and behaviors. Take time to thank people and let them know you are grateful for them. At night reflect on how fortunate you are and perhaps keep a gratitude journal to include as part of an evening prayer or meditation ritual before you go to bed.

Tapas – Willpower and Discipline

Tapas On the Mat: Think about areas in your life where you would like to develop more discipline and willpower. Visualize success in the intention of having more self-control in these areas. As you go through your physical practice, use visualizations, affirmations, mantras, positive quotes, a verse, or a prayer to reinforce that intention of developing more will power in your life—or perhaps overcoming a negative habit or harmful addiction in your life.

Tapas In the World: Practice discipline and self-control in your daily life. Build on your strengths and the things that come easy to you. Take little steps to work on your weak areas. Reinforce the positive and be gentle with yourself as you work on things that are more difficult. Use positive self-talk and even rewards for yourself to build yourself up when you are feeling challenged—and to boost your confidence as you develop more balance in your ability to discipline your thoughts, feelings, and behaviors.

Svadhyaya – Self-study and Contemplation

Svadhyaya On the Mat: Use your practice as a time to think about the things you have been studying in your life that you have read, watched, listened to or participated in. Reflect on what you have learned and perhaps what you want to learn. Set the intention to teach yourself new things and to incorporate studying into your daily life.

Svadhyaya In the World: Take time in the morning, throughout the day, and at night for personal growth and development. Find different ways to get information that is enjoyable and interesting for you. Look for things that will help you deepen understanding of something you have already been studying as well as helping you learn about new things. Find ways to do this that work with your schedule and gear up in terms of if you are more of a morning person or night person, if you learn better listening, watching or reading, and if you enjoy writing and journaling or just reflecting on things you are studying and learning. Choose user-friendly and realistic ways to make continual learning and reflecting a part of your lifestyle.

Ishvara Pranidhana – Devotion, Commitment to Spiritual Growth, and Development and Focus on Higher Good

Ishvara Pranidhana On the Mat: Take time to learn more about spirituality or your spiritual beliefs if you are a religious person. Perhaps adding prayer to your Yoga practice is a way of deepening your spiritual growth. You can also think about nature, the universe, and ways that your practice can help you to better understand yourself, others, and your community—with the intention of finding opportunities to help others as you are improving yourself.

We often say Namaste to each other in class. Namaste is saying the best or divine in me recognizes and honors the best in you. It's a sign of respect and acknowledgment. Think about ways to honor and demonstrate respect for yourself and others more.

Ishvara Pranidhana In the World: Reading sacred texts from your spiritual beliefs or other religions, attending worship services, watching videos, attending lectures and events, spending time in nature, studying science, the world, and the universe, volunteering, and being of service to others are ways you can think beyond yourself, learn about, contribute to and be a part of the greater good of life. Look for ways to lift others up.

There are many paths towards growth and enlightenment. Pick whatever works for you authentically and find ways to make this a part of your daily life.

Practicing Limb Three: *Asanas – Physical Shapes and Movements*

Asanas On the Mat: There are many styles and traditions of the physical Yoga practice that can benefit you. Depending on your physical condition and your intentions, the type of physical practice you enjoy and benefit from can be quite different for someone else.

My favorite practice is a moderate level flow, matching breath and movement. I suggest that you find a studio with certified Yoga instructors to safely develop your physical practice and get the strength and flexibility that Yoga will help you gain while avoiding injuries. Many gyms offer Yoga classes. You can also find excellent videos and articles online. There are a number of excellent books and magazines available at bookstores and online.

My favorite sequence for a physical practice is outlined at the end of this chapter. If you are interested in learning how to do these shapes and movements safely, I suggest you use a studio like Yoga Den with registered Yoga teachers and find instructions from the resources I provide at the end of this book.

Asanas In the World: As you go through your daily life, find opportunities to use these postures, movements, and shapes so you can benefit physically, emotionally, and mentally from better alignment or movements.

Often just a minor adjustment of your body will give you great results. For example, play around with mini Yoga practices when or where you want. You will find that some stretching, gentle movements and postures can help you feel more mindful, peaceful, and empowered in many situations and circumstances.

You can adapt almost any of the physical shapes and use them in many settings—from the golf course to classroom—standing or seated. You can do this sort of mini practice without anyone knowing it, drawing unwanted attention to yourself, or disturbing anyone. These micro adjustments to your posture and gentle movements of your body can be very helpful in times when you feel triggered.

Practicing Limb Four: *Pranayama – Controlled Breathing*

The following breath exercises are the most common ones that I have learned as a Yoga student, that I have used in my training, and that I use regularly as a teacher.

Pranayama On the Mat: As you center, start with bringing attention to your breath and, before you try any of the other breath exercises, just start with awareness of your breath.

Begin with slowing down, allowing yourself to relax and letting your breath bring you to the present moment. Notice the sensation of each inhalation and exhalation. Just become aware of your breath.

Start with *Dirgha* (detailed below), then shift over to *Ujjayi* (also detailed below). Continue using *Ujjayi* through your practice, and then finish your practice with whatever breath exercise you like from the list below.

Pranayama In the World: There are many opportunities to go to your breath. In many situations, you can deepen your inhalations and exhalations to feel more balanced.

If you are feeling stressed for example, you can extend your exhalations. Some of this can be done in a mixed setting without drawing any attention to yourself.

Dirgha – Three Part Breath

This deeper breath exercise of noticing your belly fill with fresh air, your chest expanding from side to side, and each inhalation rising to your collar bones as you lift your chest helps you increase lung capacity and bring more oxygen in your body.

To get comfortable with *Dirgha*, perhaps start with your hands on you belly and notice it expanding on your inhalations and contracting, as you draw navel to spine on your exhalations. You can then put your hands on each side of your ribs and notice the expansion and contractions with your breath on your chest. You can then place your hands on your collar bones and notice the air rising up towards your throat. This deeper, three-part breathing is calming for your mind, emotions, and body.

Dirgha On the Mat: This is a great breath exercise to begin your practice with, as it brings more oxygen to your body and helps you relax your mind. It is helpful to do a few rounds of this before moving on to other breath exercises and your physical practice.

Dirgha In the World: This is a great simple exercise that you can do any time you feel tense mentally or physically. You may notice that you are holding your breath or not breathing deeply as you go through your day, and this three-part breath can help you feel more mindful, peaceful, and empowered in any setting. You just need to focus and go to your breath. It is a game changer when you feel triggered. Practicing this regularly will help you in many areas of your life.

Ujjayi – *Ocean Sounding/Victorious Breath*

By constricting the back of your throat, inhaling and exhaling through your nose to make an audible ocean sound, you use your breath to calm yourself. I have heard and used the instructions many times to imaging that you are inhaling the word "ah" and exhaling the word "ha"—like you are fogging a bathroom mirror.

This breath exercise helps calm your mind and warms your body. It helps you feel both relaxed, grounded, and focused.

Ujjayi On the Mat: Shifting over to Ujjayi breath as you center and begin your practice is a great way to help you go within, relax your mind, and prepare your body for the physical asana practice. Using this breath throughout your practice will help you keep your mind calmer and your body less tense as you go through various shapes and movements.

Ujjayi In the World: This is a great breath exercise that you can do when you are feeling stressed or anxious. It helps you feel calm and focused. When I evacuated during a recent hurricane, and was in a lot of traffic leaving Florida, I used this breath to relax my mind and body—and yet say alert—while managing a tense situation.

Nadi Shodhan – Alternate Nostril Breathing

This breath exercise of inhaling through one nostril and exhaling through the other helps balance the brain's left and right hemispheres and improves concentration.

Nadi Shodhan On the Mat: Taking a few rounds of alternate nostril breathing can really help you feel grounded, cleared, balanced, and focused. I like this at the end of a practice when I'm about to go back to work or to do projects.

Nadi Shodhan In the World: This is a great breath exercise to help you feel more balanced and focused. If you are working on a project, about to take an exam, or just feeling pulled in too many directions, a few rounds of alternate nostril breathing can help you regain clarity and perspective.

Sama Vritti – Balanced Breathing

This breath exercise of inhaling through your nose, exhaling though your mouth, and pausing in between each inhalation and exhalation – all to an even count – helps to reduce stress and increase feeling of calm and balance.

Sama Vritti On the Mat: This is a great breath exercise to use when you are centering and getting grounded. You can also go to this breath if you find yourself holding tension or stress in your body during a posture. It can be a nice one to close out your practice if you are headed to work, school, or a project after you roll up your mat.

Sama Vritti In the World: This is a great breath exercise if you find yourself stressed while driving, working on a project, or in the middle of a tense situation. Since you don't need to use your hands, it's safe to go to this breath during a lot of activities, and you will likely find that you gain clarity, balance, and feel more relaxed too.

Vishama Vritti – Uneven Breath

This breath exercise of inhaling through your nose, lengthening your exhalation though your mouth, and pausing in between each inhalation and exhalation – while keeping the length of the inhalation and pause even – helps to greatly relax your mind and body.

Vishama Vritti On the Mat: This is a great breath exercise to do at the end of your practice, as it will leave you feeling calm, grounded, and very relaxed.

Vishama Vritti In the World: This is a great breath exercise to do if you are feeling agitated, overly stressed, or tense. It is incredibly calming and can be effective if you are having trouble sleeping.

Bhramari – Bumble Bee Breath

This breath exercise helps reduce agitation, anxiety, and mental tension. It is both energizing and relaxing for mind and body. There is something about doing the exhale with your lips pretty much closed and making a bumble bee sound that is a little humorous and invigorating.

Bhramari On the Mat: This is a great breath exercise for the end of your practice before you go back into the world. I find it helps lift my mood, boosts my physical energy, and clears my mind as I end a practice and go back to work or other activities.

Bhramari In the World: This is a great breath exercise if you find yourself holding tension in you jaw area because you feel stressed or uptight with yourself, others, or any given situation. Since this breath is stimulating the throat chakra area, it seems to help me with finding ways to express myself when I feel agitated and at a loss for words—or if I am tense and holding tension in my jaw. I like to use this breath to relax and improve my mood.

Practicing Limb Five: *Pratyahara – Sensory Withdrawal*

Pratyahara on the Mat. As you settle in and center let go of anything that happened before you got to your mat. Let go of anything you need to do later. Acknowledge any internal or external distractions or obstacles. Notice them without judgment and let them go. Imagine they are floating away like clouds in the sky, filing them away, or whatever image works for you.

Pratyahara In the World: As you go through your daily life, there are many obstacles and distractions that can take away from your mindfulness, peace, and empowerment. These may be internal or external and, as we acknowledge them clearly, honestly, and without judgement, we can train ourselves to let them go. The practice of sensory withdrawal is using intentional denial and compartmentalization to help us train our minds to let go of what doesn't serve us so that we can become calm—even in the midst of life's challenges.

This does not mean that we do not appropriately acknowledge and address things that need to be dealt with. It means that we take a mental step back, clear our minds, and give ourselves a mental break so that when we do focus on addressing any internal or external issues, we can do so with greater clarity, and objectivity—being more responsive and proactive and merging our intellect with our emotions, instead of being overly emotional and reactive.

As you deal with any pain, negative sensations, fears, or whatever internal or external challenges you may have, you will find that this training of your mind to go within and allowing yourself to relax and not focus on these distractions is an incredibly powerful practice.

Practicing Limb Six: *Dharana – Concentration and Focus*

Dharana On the Mat: Take a few moments as you are centering to choose something to focus and concentrate on. This can be your breath, an intention, how your body feels, an affirmation, your awareness itself, or perhaps a prayer or quote that is meaningful to you. Choose whatever comes naturally for you—and that you think will benefit you. Make that your main point of focus throughout your practice. If your mind starts to wander, or if you have stress in your body, just go back to focusing on what you've chosen as a focal point for your practice. As you train your mind to focus and concentrate on whatever you choose, you will find that internal and external obstacles and distractions essentially fall away. Learning how to concentrate and keep your focus is one of the key aspects of becoming more mindful, peaceful, and empowered. As you do this on your mat, you will learn to take this focus with you into the world.

Dharana In the World: In your daily life you get to choose what you focus on and can prioritize where your thoughts and energy go. Train your mind to concentrate on what you decide is your priority and to help remove obstacles and distractions. If you do not choose your focus, others will choose things for you focus on, and you will find your thoughts being scattered in many directions, based on what others or the media tell you to focus on.

Begin and end your days with a little time to think about what you want to focus on. Let that point of focus guide you in your choices. There will still be things that come up internally or externally that may be obstacles or distractions to your focus, but you can choose to shift your focus back on what you have prioritized. You can do this mind training in conjunction with many personal, professional, and domestic activities, and the results in terms of mental clarity are very rewarding.

Practicing Limb Seven: *Dhyana – Meditation*

Dhyana On the Mat: Allowing your mind to relax and be calm is the intention of this limb of Yoga. Some people call this stillness. Many traditions view meditation as a process that starts with sensory withdrawal and having a single point of focus to arrive at this quiet state of mind.

As you go through this process of training your mind to be calm you may find that your own thoughts or physical sensations can disrupt your quiet mind, or something external can be a distraction. This is fine and part of the process. You can simply acknowledge these obstacles or distractions to your calm and quiet mind and shift back to stillness by letting them go. It can be a somewhat fluid state and process. *Pratyahara, Dharana,* and *Dhyana* can be viewed as three levels of meditation and mind training. So, when you fall out of silence, continue using sensory withdrawal and a single point of concentration or focus to quiet your mind.

This will become easier over time. Don't get frustrated with yourself or the source of the disruption. View this as a process, like learning any skill or building muscle. You may never have a completely calm mind, but that is okay. Honor where you are, and enjoy the process. What you will find is that over time your mind will become more relaxed and calmer, and that you are able to go to this quiet place in your mind as you center and maintain this peaceful state more throughout your practice.

Dhyana In the World: There are many ways to meditate and to take the practice of concentration and stilling the mind with you throughout your daily life. A little quiet time by yourself in the morning, during your lunch break, or at night will help you develop this skill. Also, look for opportunities to make the mundane activities in your daily life into exercises in meditation. For example, yard work, dishes, laundry, driving, and any type of exercise or hobby can be a meditative practice if you use it as an opportunity to withdraw from distractions, focus, and calm your mind. This calming of the mind takes work and is incredibly rewarding.

Practicing Limb Eight: *Samadhi – Union or Bliss*

Samadhi On the Mat: Hopefully you will find moments of experiencing a sense of union or bliss or just great peace as you go through your Yoga practice. These very peaceful moments when we feel blissful, content and more connected with God or the universe—and a wonderful feeling of being both calm and empowered—are incredible to experience.

There are no shortcuts to achieving this state of heightened awareness and peacefulness. You have to work to get there. That said, there are many types of practices that will get you there. Let your energy help guide you to what level of physical and breath practice might be best for you given your mind, body, emotional, mental, and spiritual state. Sometimes the most beneficial practice for you is a slow one. Sometimes the best thing for you is more physical practice.

What is best for you varies from time to time, from season to season. There is no right or wrong practice to get you to *Samadhi*, and your Yoga practice can be in a heated room listening to rock music or very meditative in an air-conditioned studio with silence. Find the type on-the-mat-time that helps you most and be open to discovering different ways to find this state of peace. You will know it when you get there. There have times been when I could only get to this blissful state through a sun power class, and there have been times when I needed a candlelight restorative practice.

You can always choose what is best for you. There are many paths on your mat—or in a chair—to *Samadhi*.

Samadhi In the World: As you go about your daily life, you will find that some activities make you feel more of this sense of union or bliss than others and sometimes it happens when you least expect it. Pay attention to what brings you to this peaceful state. There are many paths that will bring you to *Samadhi*, but be careful not to use addictive substances such as drugs, alcohol, or activities to give you a false sense of *Samadhi*. Balance is key, and anything can be taken to excess. It seems that many of us spend our lives desperately chasing this feeling, but it also seems that the only way to really get there is through really slowing down and relaxing into the present moment.

You may find Samadhi through cooking, cleaning, walking, working, doing crossword, coloring, praying, worshiping, writing, reading, dancing, or listening to music in your car on a drive in the country or in traffic. This state of being is akin to what is called flow in happiness psychology. Be careful not to turn this into a compulsive or addictive pursuit or chase. As the saying goes, anything in excess reverses on itself, and even sunshine burns if you get too much. Strive for balance and these moments of mindfulness, peace, and empowerment will come to you and you will get to enjoy these glimpses of the divine. This is a unique experience for every person. Don't judge or compare your path with anyone else's or any other time in your life. Be who you are, find what activities you genuinely enjoy that authentically take you to Samadhi, and honor the journey—not just the destination.

Developing an Eight Limb Yoga Practice

On the Mat: As you study Yoga, work on integrating the *Yamas* and the *Niyamas* into your practice in whatever way makes sense for you. Often, during centering or at the end of your time on the mat is a good time to focus on the philosophy and then take that with you through your practice of the *Asanas, Pranayama, Pratyahara, Dhyana,* and *Dharana* and enjoying the experience of *Samadhi.*

In the World: As you go through your daily life find opportunities to practice the *Yamas, Niyamas, Asanas, Pranayama, Pratyahara, Dhyana, Dharana,* and moments of *Samadhi* so you can benefit physically, emotionally, and mentally from your practice of Yoga.

Practicing any of these aspects, or limbs, will give you great benefits—whether you are on the mat or in the world, and I hope you find ways to make Yoga a daily practice.

Going To Yoga When You Feel Challenged

You can always go to your Yoga practice when you feel triggered to help you regain mindfulness, peace, and empowerment.

Yoga is always there for you. When challenged, just realize you can use any part of Yoga to help you manage your way through whatever distractions or obstacles you are dealing with.

A Sample Asana Practice

The following is a sequence that I really enjoy for my personal practice and use in my teaching.

You can use this type of sequence for a practice as a guide to develop one of your own. Take away what doesn't work for you or add more if you want more of a challenge.

Heat up the room and make it more rigorous if you want to sweat.

Add the props like bolsters and blankets, and cut on the air conditioning to make it a very restorative practice, if that meets your needs.

As a student and teacher, I do some sort of variation of this practice on a regular basis—depending on what my energy level is, how much time I have to practice or what level class I am teaching.

To make it very simple, I view my Yoga practice in three parts: Centering; The Breathwork and Physical Shapes and Movements; The Meditative Closure. My beginning and ending are typically always the same. I just change the middle based on what I feel I need in my own practice—and what class I am teaching.

I hope this sequence is helpful to you find what benefits you too.

Play around with your practice, put on some music you like, light some candles, and have fun.

Andrew's Personal Practice

Center seated (*Lotus Pose*), set an intention, and go to your breath. Use this time to think about your relationship with yourself, others, and the world around you.

Gentle Neck Movements

Shoulder Shrugs and Rolls

Full Body Stretch on your Back

Hug Knees to Chest and Massage Back

Warm Ankles, Knees, and Hips

Roll Up to Seated

Seated Spinal Twist

Side Stretches

Table (*Bharmanasana*)

Cat (*Marjyasana*) and Cow (*Bitilasana*)

Thread The Needle (*Parsva Balasana*)

Spinal Balance (*Dandayamna Bharmanasana*)

Puppy Stretch (*Uttana Shishosana*)

Downward Dog (*Adho Mukha Svanasana)*

Forward Fold (*Uttanasana*)

Gentle Standing Back Bend (*Anuvittasana*)

Mountain (*Tadasana*)

Crescent of Half Moon (*Urdhva Hastasana*)

Tree (*Vrksasana)*

Sun Salutation A (*Surya Namaskara A)*

Chair (*Utkatasana*)

Chair Twist/ Revolved Chair Pose (*Parivrtta Utkatasana*)

Sun Salutation B (*Surya Namaskara)*

Warrior I (*Virabhadrasana I*)

Warrior II (*Virabhadrasana II*)

Extended Side Angle (*Parsvakonasana*)

Triangle (*Trikonasana*)

Pyramid (*Parsvottanasana*)

Warrior III (*Virabhadrasana III*)

Three Point Balance

Half Moon (*Adha Chandrasana*)

Revolved Half Moon (*Parivrtta Ardha Chandrasana*)

Wild Thing (*Camatkarasana*) Feel free to flip your dog!

Plank

Side Plank (*Vasisthasana*)

Thread the Needle in Side Plank

Cobra (<u>Bhujangasana</u>)

Child's Pose (*Balasana)*

Pigeon (*Eka Pada Rajakapotasana*)

Bound Angle (*Baddha Konasana*)

Full or Double Pigeon (*Agnistambhasana*)

Staff Pose (*Dandasana*)

Seated Spinal Twist or Half Lord of the Fishes Pose (*Matsyendrasana*)

Head-to-Knee Forward Fold (*Janu Sirsasana*)

Forward Seated Fold/Posterior Stretch (*Paschimottanasana*)

Upward Facing Boat (*Navasana*)

Bridge (Setu Bandha Sarvangasana)

Knees-to-Chest Post (*Apanasana*) *Give Yourself a Hug!*

Half Shoulder Stand (*Ardha Sarvangasana*) or other Inversion, as restorative or advanced as you enjoy

Happy Baby (*Ananda Balasana*)

Alternate Knees to Chest (*Apanasana*)

Supine Spinal Twist (*Supta Matsyendrasana*) ending in Supine Tree in Each Direction

Take a full body stretch.

Get comfortable with a bolster under your knees or upper back, a blanket, or whatever feels best for you.

Do a Yoga Nidra relaxation of your whole body from your toes to your head.

Chakra's Meditation: Bring your attention to Brow Area, Third Eye Chakra. Gaze into darkness. Visualize Colors: Red, Orange, Yellow, Green, Blue, and White.

White Light Healing Meditation: Imagine there's a white light above the crown of your head, swirling round and round, a healing white light, moving slowly down your face, neck and shoulders, arms and torso, down your legs to the bottom of your feet, a healing warm white light, permeating every cell and fiber of your body.

Corpse Pose (*Savasana*)

Reawaken your body with gentle movements, brush your thumbs across your fingertips, wiggle your toes, and roll your head some from side to side. Roll over onto your side, curl into self, and just enjoy a few moments here. Then, with your eyes closed, press into your mat with your palms, and let your senses guide you back to Seated (Lotus).

Closing Breath Exercise (I typically like *Vishama Vritti.*)

Bring your arms along your side body, inhale your hands up and together, pausing in the following ways as a closing sequence:

Hands to Forehead as a reminder that Yoga creates space in our minds—space between stimuli, our thoughts, emotions, bodies, and behaviors—choosing with intent, responding instead of reacting;

Hands to eyes as a reminder that through Yoga we see ourselves, others, and the world around us with clearer vision, kind eyes, and compassion;

Hands to mouth as a reminder that we can always give the gift of Karma Yoga—a smile, kind words, and encouragement—speaking your truth, knowing your boundaries; and

Hands to heart as a reminder that Yoga is more than a physical practice and that we are cultivating balance—mind, body, and spirit.

Bring your intention back to the forefront of your mind, visualize it clearly again, and carry your intention with you as you roll up your mat and go back in the world.

With Love and Gratitude, Namaste

Chapter Four: Integrated Daily Practice

"Your daily life is your temple and your religion. When you enter into it take with you your all."

Khalil Gibran

"Day by day, what you choose, what you think and what you do is who you become."

Heraclitus

Integrated Daily Practice

Bringing elements of Meta-Awareness, Framing, and Yoga together in your daily life will help you become more mindful, peaceful, and empowered. I suggest you use your dedicated times each day for these practices to explore how they connect and what works for you. I also hope that when you find yourself triggered by any internal or external stimuli, that you will find ways to go to all three of these practices to help you work through challenges.

As you develop an integrated daily practice, you will become more responsive and proactive—instead of reactive, and you will improve the alignment of your thoughts and actions to be more congruent with your intentions, values, and spiritual beliefs through these practices.

You will find how to best work times to practice Meta-Awareness, Framing, and Yoga in your life, and they don't have to take long. Setting aside a few blocks of time that can be only five to fifteen minutes to dedicate to these practices will yield large results for you in terms of becoming more mindful, peaceful, and empowered.

As you begin learning to intentionally develop the skill of creating space between stimuli and responding—choosing with intent, responding instead of reacting—some of the parts of Meta-Awareness, Framing, and Yoga will come easier to you than others. You will find what works best for you by taking time to just play around with applying these concepts in your daily life.

You will also start to notice that there are many opportunities in your daily life to go to Meta-Awareness, Framing, and Yoga and use parts of them to either enhance what is going well in your life—or to help you manage times when you are feeling challenged and reactive by internal or external triggers.

Integrated Daily Practice Helps You Cultivate Mindfulness, Peace, and Empowerment

As you engage in the Mindfulness practice of Meta-Awareness you will gain a greater level of clarity of your awareness itself, your thoughts, your emotions, your body, your behaviors, your relationships with yourself, others and the world around you. You will notice how your choices are either congruent or incongruent with your intentions, values, and spiritual beliefs—and whether the thoughts and behaviors you choose are working for or working against you in your intent to have more mindfulness, peace, and empowerment in your life. You will notice (without judgment) ways in which you are and are not where you want to be, how you want to be, and who you want to be. You will gain a better understanding of your strengths and weaknesses. You will see which distractions, obstacles, and triggers impact you the most in terms of taking away from mindfulness, peace, and empowerment.

This level of clarity may feel very uncomfortable at first, and a big part of these practices is to focus on that awareness, and sit with the discomfort you notice. By engaging with reality instead of avoiding it, you will find that some things in your life that you may need to accept, and just do nothing at all. Just noticing may be enough at times.

At other times you will determine that the best choice is to take some type of action to address the areas of discomfort. This will usually be the case, as action can simply be shifting your thoughts or stopping thinking about or doing something. This does not have to involve direct engagement with anyone. Yoga philosophy, the physical practice, breathwork and meditative techniques will help you with this personal journal.

From Awareness you can choose what you want to do with Framing and Yoga and let your personal growth and development be the motivation—not external feedback or the opinions of others. As you work with the practices of Meta-Awareness, Framing, and Yoga, and you notice things that are challenging, you may find that the practice of just acknowledging and allowing the thoughts and feelings, as well as sensations in your body, to pass over time.

There are some challenges that we can't rush through or avoid, such as grief and disappointment. If you find that you're keeping your mind or body active as a way to avoid and not acknowledge something painful, you will find that there is really no way around addressing difficult truths. Often what we suppress grows and becomes even more challenging because of avoidance. Learning to be aware of even the unpleasant aspects of our own psyche and life experiences can help us become stronger and more resilient just by having the courage to face and work through harsh realities.

Some things you just have to go through and accept—without taking any big steps in terms of shifting your thoughts or behaviors, and going through these things with awareness and humility can give you something to feel proud of once you've gone through them. At other times, you will realize that the healthiest choice in responding to a challenge is to take some sort of appropriate action in shifting your thoughts and behaviors as you seek to improve your relationships with yourself, others, and the world around you.

You will find this greater level of clarity and intent by using Framing to improve on what and how you focus externally—and then being better guided in how you choose to engage with other and the world around you is a powerful way to align or realign your thoughts and behaviors with your intentions and reality.

You may find it easier to be clearer, kinder, and more direct with people you have had trouble communicating effectively with in the past. You may also find that following the instructions provided in Yoga, its philosophy, the physical exercise and postures, the breath work, and the mind training will help you have more compassion, strength, and efficacy in how you relate with others and better engage with the world around you.

For example, if traffic and aggressive and distracted drivers are something that you find really aggravating, you may be better able to step back emotionally and not react to others' reckless behavior by just focusing, clearing your mind, and responding with skill and capability as a driver—without having an unnecessary emotional overlay that typically does not serve any of us well. You will still be engaged appropriately with the thoughts and behaviors needed to drive defensively and safely, but you will find less stress in your body and mind as you work with your alignment—focusing on what is in your control, and perhaps have some sympathy and compassion for those who are acting in such a foolish way. The process is simple: (1) notice you're triggered; (2) go to whatever aspects of Meta-Awareness, Framing, and Yoga serve you in that circumstance; and (3) use those practices to make healthier choices in your thoughts and behaviors. Then check in again, and repeat as needed.

As you engage in the powerful practice of Framing you will gain a greater level of clarity from choosing what you focus on how, and refocusing and shifting your perspective as needed. This Framing and Reframing process will help you have more positive and clear thoughts, more balanced emotions, improved feelings in your body—in terms of holding less stress and tension, and better and internal external outcomes from how you relate in your communications.

As you work Framing and Re-framing and become more intentional and disciplined with what you think about and how you think, you will probably experience clearer and less emotionally charged thinking, you'll feel more balanced and temperate in your thoughts and behaviors, and your experience of mindfulness, peace, and empowerment will increase as you are aligning your thoughts and behaviors with your intentions, values, and spiritual beliefs, your awareness will increase as you work with Framing, and this awareness leads you to better choices.

As you practice Yoga (on and off the mat) you will experience many mental, physical, emotional, and spiritual benefits. While these benefits and results of your practice will be different from anyone else's, you will find that as you gain strength and flexibility in your body, you will also gain strength and flexibility in your mind. This leads to feeling more mindful and the ability to manage your life from peaceful and empowered place. Regardless of what type of Yoga practice you develop, you will experience benefits from the practice of any or all the eight limbs of Yoga. Any Yoga is Yoga.

You may find that through Yoga practice you increase your awareness and that the concept and practice of Meta-Awareness ties in quite naturally with your Yoga practice.
As you practice Yoga, you can make it an intention to focus on your awareness and mindfully observe your awareness.
This deeper level of awareness, intuition, inner wisdom—whatever term you have for it—will lead you to clearer understanding and assessments of your thoughts, your emotions, your body, your behaviors, and your relationship with yourself, others, and the world around you.
You will notice where your choices are in alignment with your intentions and values—and which ones are out of alignment.

As you see how you manage your time, energy, money and the outcomes of your choices more clearly, you can make minor readjustments as needed in your choice of thoughts and behaviors to guide you more towards who you want to be and how you want your life to be.

This process happens naturally because Yoga is a training of the mind and body that yields great spiritual growth and improvement in our relationships with self and others.

The instructions and exercises in the eight limbs of Yoga lead to mindfulness, peace and empowerment.

You may also find that through Yoga you gain a better understanding of how you Frame your life, others, experiences and events. Your active mind may create more noise than usual as you start to practice Yoga.

This resistance in the form of excessive mind chatter can be very insightful because you can use what you notice regarding your mind activity as a better way to understand what your mind is focused on, how it is perceiving things, and what you can improve on. You may find a lot of things from the past come up, perhaps fears about the future, perhaps negative judgments about yourself and others.

Perhaps even judgment that you should be doing something more "productive" with the time you are spending practicing Yoga. You may be surprised by the thoughts and emotions that come up during a physical practice on the mat and by being more engaged mentally as you are in the world doing your practice. You can use the noticing of these thoughts and emotions to become more deliberate and intentional with your Yoga practice and how you Frame and Reframe reality in your daily life—on and off the mat.

As you find ways in your daily life to set aside dedicated time to work with and enjoy the practices of Meta-Awareness, Framing, and Yoga, you will discover what works best for you and your schedule on a daily or weekly basis.

Some of these practices will seem natural and come easier to you and provide you quickly with benefits in terms of cultivating mindfulness, peace, and empoweremnt in your life. Other parts of this may take a bit more work to develop ways to practice the concepts and activities and then apply them naturally as you go through your life experiences.

You will find ways to practice Meta-Awareness, Framing and Yoga as a part of your daily life and regular life activities and responsibilities.

These practices can become an integrated and sustainable part of your lifestyle—not just things you do when you have extra time. And you can always go to these practices at any time you need them.

There is no right or wrong way or order to doing these practices. Just start to do what works for you. We are all different and each day is different. Don't compare yourself with anyone one else or with any other time in your life as you start making these practices a part of your daily routine. Don't judge yourself. Notice whatever comes up in your thoughts, emotions, body, behaviors, and acknowledge it as a way of gaining better understanding—not to beat yourself up in any way about how you should be, or how you once were. Honor where you are, and be present with these practices and how they affect you.

These practices are certainly not some sort of magic cure-all for whatever you may feel is wrong, missing, or out of alignment in your life, but they do work and get you incredible results in all areas of your life if you are willing to do them on a regular basis. I have found that these practices have helped me work thought many minor and major internal and external distractions, obstacles, and triggers that include body image, relationships with family, friends, colleagues, compulsive and impulsive tendencies, and healing from past traumas—and having more confidence, feelings of security in the present, and hope for the future.

These practices have certainly helped me create space between exposure to stimuli and how I respond. I'm still affected emotionally when I hear news of a mass shooting, see upsetting political discourse on social media, feel ill, get a letter from the IRS, am cut off or tailgated by an aggressive driver, or someone is rude to me. However, I tend to now step back and notice what is going on—go to Meta-Awareness, Framing, and Yoga, in some way or combination of parts of these three practices that make sense in the moment—and respond instead of reacting and am intentional with my thoughts and behaviors.

While it sounds obvious—and is certainly common sense—practicing the pause and creating space to align our thoughts with our intentions, values, and spiritual beliefs takes work. Some triggers like physical or emotional pain, the news of a loved one's illness or death, or an argument with someone you care about can throw any of us off. Many of us have some sort of established patterns of reacting instead of responding and being somewhat mindless with our thoughts and behaviors. We also have many strengths and positive patterns to build on as we become more mindful.

As I've learned to pause and create space before I respond, I have improved my ability of aligning my thoughts and behaviors with my intentions values, and spiritual beliefs, and I have experienced more mindfulness, peace, and empowerment.

As a person who has often been very reactive and unaware of the fact that I had choices, this shift in not just how I perceive my life, but how I now live, is a huge improvement to say the least. I still fall out of balance and am challenged on a regular basis by focusing on my own weaknesses and on things that are beyond my control in the world around me. But through these daily practices I have learned to better manage my thoughts, emotions, and behaviors and enjoy a happier and healthier life. I hope you find that these practices provide you with similar positive results in your life.

Creating The Space Between Worksheet

What are stimuli that can be a distraction, obstacle, or trigger for you?

What is your typical reactive pattern to this stimulus? What are reactive thoughts and behaviors triggered by this stimulus that take you away from mindfulness, peace, and empowerment?

What are the outcomes of these reactive thoughts and behaviors? How do they affect your thoughts, emotions, body, behaviors, relationships with yourself, others, and the world around you? What are the short and long-term results and consequences of being reactive?

Stepping back as a nonjudgmental observer, how can you use Meta-Awareness more quickly identify when you are feeling triggered and to make healthier proactive and responsive choices in terms of your thoughts and behaviors when you are triggered by this stimulus?

Based on this assessment, how could you handle things better? What thoughts and behaviors are more congruent and in alignment with your intentions, values, and spiritual beliefs?

How do you think these improved proactive and responsive choices would affect your How do they affect your thoughts, emotions, body, behaviors, relationships with yourself, others, and the world around you?

How can you improve the way you handle this trigger with Framing?

How does what you are focusing on affect you?

How does the amount of energy you spending on focusing on things (the news, fears, the past, the future, others, etc.) affect you?

How does the way you focus affect you?

Can you reframe and shift your focus?

What parts of Yoga would help you when exposed to this stimulus?

Yamas: How are you treating other and acting towards them?

Nijamas: How are you treating yourself and acting towards yourself and who you want to be?

Breathwork: what breath exercise can you go to? Are you breathing mindfully and deeply (three part)? What else works for you in this situation?

Asansa: something physical on any level, on or off your mat, depending on the circumstance and trigger.

Sensory Withdrawal can you step back from the trigger or the pattern or obstacle or habit and disengage some in terms of thoughts and behaviors. Imaging it's floating away, file it away as an exercises in intentional denial or compartmentalization.

Focus: can you focus then on an intention, your values, your spiritual beliefs, a mantra, an aspect of your awareness or framing to train your mind and you attend to something other than the obstacle and instead bring it to the forefront of your mind?

Meditation: can you calm your mind and just find a sense of peace within yourself—even if something significant is triggering you internally or externally?

Samadhi: Can you find bliss in the midst of this? Can you work through this challenge and transcend it?

When this happens evaluate how you did? What improved? What was still a challenge for you?

Repeat

Keep building on what is working well for you and adjusting what needs improvement with the help of Meta-Awareness, Framing, and Yoga.

Notes

Chapter One: Meta-Awareness

The concept of the real you being the one that notices was introduced to me in the book, *The Untethered Soul: The Journey Beyond Yourself* by Michael A. Singer:
https://www.amazon.com/Untethered-Soul-Journey-Beyond-Yourself/dp/1572245379

I first read about the idea of having a higher level of thinking or greater mind ability in the book. *The Power of Now: A Guide to Spiritual Enlightenment:* https://www.amazon.com/Power-Now-Guide-Spiritual-Enlightenment-ebook/dp/B002361MLA by Eckhart Tolle

Brené Brown discusses taking an honest look at our weak areas as a way of gaining strength in her Ted Talk, *The Power of Vulnerability:* https://www.ted.com/talks/brene_brown_on_vulnerability

My friend Cindy Flynn has an expression that sums up the power of clarity and my approach to this work. She says, "Name it, Claim It, and Move on." This succinctly states a way to use your awareness of internal and external stimuli that you are reactive to as a way of moving forward with intent.

One of my first introductions to identifying and overcoming negative thinking was the work of Dr. Wayne W. Dyer. His groundbreaking book *Your Erroneous Zones* helped launch his career, and much of his work has helped personally and professionally.

Your Erroneous Zones: Step-by-Step Advice for Escaping the Trap of Negative Thinking and Taking Control of Your Life by Wayne Dyer: https://www.amazon.com/Your-Erroneous-Zones-Step-Step/dp/0060919760/ref=sr_1_3?s=books&ie=UTF8&qid=1539316370&sr=1-3&keywords=wayne+dyer+books

The Power of Intention by Dr. Wayne W. Dyer:
https://www.amazon.com/Power-Intention-Dr-Wayne-Dyer/dp/1401902162/ref=sr_1_4?s=books&ie=UTF8&qid=1539316552&sr=1-4&keywords=wayne+dyer+books

The Miracle of Mindfulness: An Introduction to the Practice of Meditation by Thich Nhat Hanh: https://www.amazon.com/Miracle-Mindfulness-Introduction-Practice-Meditation/dp/0807012394/ref=sr_1_1?s=books&ie=UTF8&qid=1539400598&sr=1-1&keywords=the+miracle+of+mindfulness+by+thich+nhat+hanh

Don't Bite the Hook: Finding Freedom from Anger, Resentment, and Other Destructive Emotions by Pema Chodron:
https://www.amazon.com/Dont-Bite-Hook-Resentment-Destructive/dp/B077VX1HSD/ref=sr_1_16?ie=UTF8&qid=1539400734&sr=1-16&keywords=pema+chodron

The Post-Traumatic Stress Disorder Sourcebook: A Guide to Healing, Recovery by Glenn R. Schiraldi, Ph.D.

Overwhelmed: Coping with Life's Ups and Downs by Nancy K. Schlossberg:
https://www.amazon.com/gp/product/1590771265/ref=dbs_a_def_rwt_hsch_vapi_taft_p1_i3

Wherever You Go, There You Are: Mindfulness Meditation in Everyday Life by Jon Kabat-Zinn:
https://www.amazon.com/Wherever-You-There-Are-Mindfulness/dp/1401307787/ref=sr_1_1?s=books&ie=UTF8&qid=1539400523&sr=1-1&keywords=whereever+you+go+there+you+are+by+jon+kabat-zinn

Codependent No More: How to Stop Controlling Others and Start Caring for Yourself by Melody Beattie:
https://www.amazon.com/Codependent-No-More-Controlling-Yourself/dp/0894864025/ref=sr_1_9?s=books&ie=UTF8&qid=1539400113&sr=1-9&keywords=The+Language+of+Letting+Go

As I have worked observe and evaluate my thoughts, I have found it helpful to identify cognitive disorders that lead me away from mindfulness, peace, and empowerment and oven lead to reactive thoughts, emotions, and behaviors.

Ten common cognitive distortions identified by Burns are: All or Nothing Thinking, Overgeneralization, Mental Filter, Discounting the Positive, Jumping to Conclusions, Magnification of Minimalization, Emotional Reasoning, Should Statements, Labeling, and Personalization and Blame.

A cognitive distortion checklist and worksheet is available at: https://www.apsu.edu/sites/apsu.edu/files/counseling/COGNITIVE_0.pdf.

"10 Cognitive Distortions" by Therese Borchard https://www.everydayhealth.com/columns/therese-borchard-sanity-break/10-cognitive-distortions/

"Fifteen Ways To Untwist Your Thinking" by David D. Burns, M.D.: http://cognitivetherapymd.com/Links/Fifteen.htm

"Depression and Ruminative Thinking" by Madeline R. Vann, MPH: https://www.everydayhealth.com/depression/depression-and-ruminative-thinking.aspx

Feeling Good: The New Mood Therapy by David Burns, M.D.: https://www.amazon.com/Feeling-Good-The-Mood-Therapy/dp/0380810336

When Panic Attacks: The New, Drug-Free Anxiety Therapy That Can Change Your Life by David Burns, M.D.: https://www.amazon.com/When-Panic-Attacks-Drug-Free-Anxiety/dp/076792083X/ref=pd_lpo_sbs_14_t_2?_encoding=UTF8&psc=1&refRID=CXTGB4WRBSJADERTFSH6

Another great resource that I find helpful regarding emotional awareness is the work by Daniel Goldman:

Emotional Intelligence: Why It Can Matter More Than IQ:
https://www.amazon.com/gp/product/055338371X/ref=dbs_a_def_r
wt_bibl_vppi_i0

"Emotional Intelligence:"
http://www.danielgoleman.info/topics/emotional-intelligence/

My work and personal growth have been informed by my researching the work of Howard Gardner who is a pioneer in the field of intelligence and creativity. As you work to identify your strengths and to think smarter, not harder, you may find his research accessible and helpful.

His theory of Multiple Intelligences identifies the following types of intelligence: Linguistic intelligence ("word smart"), Logical-mathematical intelligence ("number/reasoning smart"), Spatial intelligence ("picture smart"), Bodily-Kinesthetic intelligence ("body smart"), Musical intelligence ("music smart"), Interpersonal intelligence ("people smart"), Intrapersonal intelligence ("self smart"), and Naturalist intelligence ("nature smart"). Source: "A Beginner's Guide to the Theory of Multiple Intelligences:" http://multipleintelligencesoasis.org/about/

Frames of Mind: The Theory of Multiple Intelligences by Howard Gardner: https://www.amazon.com/Frames-Mind-Theory-Multiple-Intelligences/dp/0465024335/ref=sr_1_2?s=books&ie=UTF8&qid=1539313184&sr=1-2&keywords=howard+gardner+multiple+intelligences

Intelligence Reframed: Multiple Intelligences for the 21ist Century by Howard Gardner:
https://www.amazon.com/dp/0465026117/ref=sxbs_sxwds-stvpv2_1?pf_rd_m=ATVPDKIKX0DER&pf_rd_p=6375e697-f226-4dbd-a63a-5ec697811ee1&pd_rd_wg=sxmk3&pf_rd_r=NFAF9RMXZHBNBCB32EGK&pf_rd_s=desktop-sx-bottom-slot&pf_rd_t=301&pd_rd_i=0465026117&pd_rd_w=chBCQ&pf_rd_i=null&pd_rd_r=4ab1d1c0-c559-4fd4-9c9e-954624bbc992&ie=UTF8&qid=1539313447&sr=1

As part of my 300 Hour Advanced Teacher Training, I studied Ayurveda and the Doshas with Dr. Jon Repole and Heather Fisse this helped me have a greater body awareness and awareness of some of my predispositions in terms of thoughts and behavioral patterns.

Ayurveda: The Science of Self Healing by Dr. Vasant Lad:
https://www.amazon.com/Ayurveda-Science-Healing-Practical-Guide/dp/0914955004/ref=sr_1_10?s=books&ie=UTF8&qid=15393 15203&sr=1-10&keywords=aryuveda+books

I was also first introduced to the idea of the Chakras and our Energy Body in work by Carolyne Myss. I found her books and audios very helpful in understanding how I held stress in my body and continue to use what I learned from her personally and professionally.

"Chakras: Your Energetic Being" by Caroline Myss:
https://www.myss.com/free-resources/chakras-your-energetic-being/

Anatomy of the Spirit: The Seven Stages of Power and Healing by Caroline Myss: https://www.amazon.com/Anatomy-Spirit-Seven-Stages-Healing/dp/0609800140/ref=sr_1_1?s=books&ie=UTF8&qid=1539 315406&sr=1-1&keywords=caroline+myss

Advanced Energy Anatomy: The Science of Co-Creation and Your Power of Choice by Caroline Myss:
https://www.amazon.com/Advanced-Energy-Anatomy-Science-Co-Creation/dp/B00006393R/ref=sr_1_7?ie=UTF8&qid=1539315406&sr=1-7&keywords=caroline+myss

The Four Agreements: A Practical Guide to Personal Freedom (A Toltec Wisdom Book) by Don Miguel Ruiz
https://www.amazon.com/Four-Agreements-Practical-Personal-Freedom/dp/1878424319/ref=sr_1_1?s=books&ie=UTF8&qid=1539 315322&sr=1-1&keywords=the+four+agreements

Mindfulness: An Eight-Week Plan for Finding Peace in a Frantic World by Mark Williams and Danny Penman: https://www.amazon.com/Mindfulness-Eight-Week-Finding-Peace-Frantic/dp/1609618955/ref=sr_1_4?s=books&ie=UTF8&qid=1539314902&sr=1-4&keywords=mindfulness

Mindfulness on the Go Cards: 52 Simple Meditation Practices You Can Do Anywhere by Jan Chozen Bays: https://www.amazon.com/Mindfulness-Go-Cards-Meditation-Practices/dp/1611803705/ref=sr_1_4?s=books&ie=UTF8&qid=1539315125&sr=1-4&keywords=mindfulness+on+the+go

Chapter Two: Framing

In her seminal book, *A Return To Love: Reflections on the Principle of A Course in Miracles*, Marianne Williamson discusses a shift in perspective being a miracle: https://www.amazon.com/Return-Love-Reflections-Principles-Miracles-ebook/dp/B000VYX944

I have been greatly influenced by much of Marianne Williamson's body of work. I spend many hours listening to her audio cassettes during my undergraduate education, her CD's during my graduate school years, and continued to listen to her work as MP3 files and on my Audible app. I continue to use a lot of the things I learned from her teaching in my writing, teaching Yoga, and personally.

The Tao of Pooh by Benjamin Hoff: https://www.amazon.com/Tao-Pooh-Benjamin-Hoff/dp/0140067477/ref=sr_1_1?ie=UTF8&qid=1539316655&sr=8-1&keywords=tao+of+pooh+book

The Red Shoes: On Torment and Recovery of Soul Life by Clarissa Pinkola Estes: https://www.amazon.com/s/ref=nb_sb_ss_i_1_15?url=search-alias%3Daps&field-keywords=red+shoes+by+estes&sprefix=red+shoes+estes%2Caps%2C228&crid=36GLMYQG738HV

The idea of looking at your storyline and seeing how it is working is one I encountered in the book, *The Law of Attraction: The Basics of the Teachings of Abraham* by Esther Hicks: https://www.amazon.com/Law-Attraction-Basics-Teachings-Abraham/dp/1401912273.

Howard Gardener

Using Affirmation books in the morning and at night can help you frame your life the way you want it to be, set your own agenda, and prime yourself to focus on what is important to you. Some of my favorites include:

The idea of learning to look at things in our live—and ourselves— more archetypally was influenced by the work of Caroline Myss and Joseph Campbell

Archetype Cards by Caroline Myss: https://www.amazon.com/Archetype-Cards-Caroline-Myss/dp/1401901840/ref=sr_1_4?s=books&ie=UTF8&qid=153931 5406&sr=1-4&keywords=caroline+myss

The Language of Archetypes: Discover the Forces that Shape Your Destiny by Caroline Myss: https://www.amazon.com/Language-Archetypes-Discover-Forces-Destiny/dp/B000I2KQ8G/ref=sr_1_21?ie=UTF8&qid=1539315645 &sr=1-21&keywords=caroline+myss
Three Levels of Power and How to Use Them by Caroline Myss: https://www.amazon.com/Three-Levels-Power-Caroline-Myss/dp/B003HRRCEU/ref=sr_1_cc_1?s=aps&ie=UTF8&qid=153 9315727&sr=1-1-catcorr&keywords=caroline+myss+three+levels+of+power

The Hero with a Thousand Faces (The Collected Works of Joseph Campbell) by Joseph Campbell:
https://www.amazon.com/s/ref=nb_sb_ss_fb_1_16?url=search-alias%3Dstripbooks&field-keywords=joseph+campbell+hero+with+a+thousand+faces&sprefix=joseph+campbell+%2Cdigital-music%2C265&crid=2VBQIEVD6JYDA

The Power of Myth by Joseph Campbell with Bill Moyers:
https://www.amazon.com/Power-Myth-Joseph-Campbell/dp/0385418868/ref=sr_1_3?s=books&ie=UTF8&qid=1539315843&sr=1-3&keywords=joseph+campbell+hero+with+a+thousand+faces

The Archetypes and The Collective Unconscious (Collected Works of C.G. Jung Vol.9 Part 1) by C. G. Jung (Author) and R.F.C. Hull (Translator)

The Faithful Gardener: A Wise Tale About That Which Can Never Die by Clarissa Pin Estes: https://www.amazon.com/Faithful-Gardener-About-Which-Never/dp/006251380X/ref=sr_1_4?s=books&ie=UTF8&qid=1539316135&sr=1-4&keywords=clarissa+pinkola+est%C3%A9s

Mother Night: Myths, Stories and Teachings for Learning to See in the Dark by Clarissa Pinkola Estes:
https://www.amazon.com/Mother-Night-Stories-Teachings-Learning/dp/B0037MA84G/ref=sr_1_5?ie=UTF8&qid=1539316189&sr=1-5&keywords=clarissa+pinkola+est%C3%A9s

The Gift of Story: A Wise Tale About What is Enough by Clarissa Pinkola Estes: https://www.amazon.com/Gift-Story-Wise-About-Enough/dp/0345388356/ref=sr_1_18?s=books&ie=UTF8&qid=1539316284&sr=1-18&keywords=clarissa+pinkola+est%C3%A9s

Creative Visualization: Use the Power of Your Imagination to Create What You Want in Your Life Paperback by Shakti Gawain: https://www.amazon.com/Creative-Visualization-Power-Imagination-Create/dp/1577312295

Power Thoughts: 12 Strategies to Win the Battle of the Mind by
Joyce Meyer: https://www.amazon.com/Power-Thoughts-
Strategies-Battle-
Mind/dp/1455504378/ref=sr_1_1?ie=UTF8&qid=1531583236&sr
=8-1&keywords=power+thoughts+joyce+meyer

My use of Framing Theory as a practice to help cultivate
mindfulness, peace and empowerment has grown out of my work
with this theory as a scholar. I first became interested in it during my
doctoral studies at University of Florida in a Graduate Seminar
taught by Dr. Spiro Kiousis and developed my dissertation under the
supervision of my late mentor and friend Dr. Lynda Kee Kaid. I
continued to use Framing as a theoretical underpinning for my
research when I was a professor at Virginia Tech where I taught
graduate seminars about Framing, Agenda Setting, and Priming to
MA students in Communication. Second level agenda setting, Meta-
communication, These three closely- related Theories inform my
perspective on applying Framing and Reframing in our lives. If you
are interested in reading more about these theories, below is a list of
seminal literature that I taught, researched, and scholarship I worked
on myself:

Berger, B.K. (2001). Private issues and public policy: Locating the
corporate agenda in agenda-setting. Journal of Public Relations
Research, 13 (2), 91-126.

Boyle, Thomas P. (2001). "Intermedia Agenda Setting in the 1996
Presidential Election." Journalism and Mass Communication
Quarterly, Vol. 78, No. 1, Spring 2001, pp. 26-44.

Chyi, Hsiang Iris and McCombs, Maxwell (2004). Media salience
and the process of framing: Coverage of the Columbine school
shooting. Journalism and Mass Communication Quarterly 81 (1), 22-
35.

Cohen, B. (1963). The press and foreign policy. Princeton, NJ:
Princeton University Press.

Constantinescu, A., & Tedesco, J. C. (2007). Framing a kidnapping: Frame convergence between online newspaper coverage and reader discussion posts about three kidnapped Romanian journalists. Journalism Studies, 8(3), 444-464.

De Vreese, Claes H., Peter Jochen, and Semetko, Holli A. (2001). Framing politics at the launch of the Euro: A cross-national comparative study of frames in the news. Political Communication 18, 107-122.

Dimitrova. D.V., Kaid, L.L., & Williams, A.P. (2004). The First Hours of the War: Online News Coverage of Operation Iraqi Freedom in R.D. Berenger (Ed.) Global Media Go to War (pp. 255-264). Spokane, WA: Marquette Books.

Dimitrova, D.V., Kaid, L. L., Williams, A.P, & Trammell, K. D. (2005). War on the Web: The immediate news framing of Gulf War II. The Harvard International Journal of Press/Politics (10)1, 22-24.

Danielian, Lucig H., & Reese, Stephen, D. (1989). A Closer Look at Intermedia Influences on Agenda Setting: The cocaine Issue of 1986. Communication Campaigns About Drugs, Government, Media and the Public, ed. Shoemaker, Pamela J. Hillsdale, JH: Lawrence Erlbaum Associates.

Funkhouser, G.R. (1973). The issues of the sixties: An exploratory study of the dynamics of public opinion. Public Opinion Quarterly, 37, 72-75.

Gandy, O. H. (1982). Beyond agenda setting: Information subsidies and public policy. Norwood, NJ: Ablex.

Ghanem, Salma (1997). Filling in the tapestry: The second level of agenda setting. In Maxwell McCombs, Donald L. Shaw and David Weaver (eds.) Communication in Democracy: Exploring the Intellectual Frontiers in Agenda-Setting Theory. Mahwah, NJ: Lawrence Erlbaum Associates, 3-14.

Golan, Guy and Wanta, Wayne (2001). Second-level agenda setting in the New Hampshire primary: A comparison of coverage in three newspapers and public perceptions of candidates. Journalism and Mass Communication Quarterly 8 (2), 247-259.

Gunther, Albert C. (1998). The persuasive press inference: Effects of mass media on perceived public opinion. Communication Research 25 (5), 486-504.

Hallahan, K. (1999). "Seven models of framing: Implications for public relations." Journal of Public Relations Research 11(3): 205-242.

Kim, S., Scheufele, D. A., & Shanahan, James (2002). Think About It This Way: Attribute Agenda-Setting Function Of The Press And The Public's Evaluation Of A Local Issue. Journalism & Mass Communication Quarterly, Vol. 79, No. 1, Spring 2002, pp. 7-25.

Kiousis, S., Bantimaroudis, P. & Ban, H. (1999). Candidate Image Attributes: experiments on the substantive dimension of second-level agenda setting. Communication Research, 26, 414-428.

Iyengar, Shanto and Kinder, Donald R. (1987). The agenda-setting effect. News that matters: Television and American Opinion, Chicago, IL: University of Chicago Press, pp. 16-33.

Iyengar, Shanto (1996). Agenda setting and beyond: Television News and strength of political issues. Riker, William H (ed.) Agenda Formation. Ann Arbor: University of Michigan Press, pp. 211-229.

Kaid, L. L. (1976). Newspaper treatment of a candidate's news releases. Journalism Quarterly, 53, 135-137.

Kaid, L.L., Hale, K., & Williams, J. (1977). Media agenda-setting of aspecific political event. Journalism Quarterly, 54, 584-587.

Kaid, L.L., Postelnicu, M., Landreville, K.D., Williams, A. P., Hostrup-Larsen, C., Urriste, S., Fernandes, J., Yun, H.J., & Bagley, A. (2005). Campaigning in the New Europe: News Media Presentations of the 2004 European Union Parliamentary Elections. In C. Holtz-Bacha (Ed.), Europawahl 2004: Massenmedien im Europawahlkampf (European Vote 2004: The Mass Media in the European Election Campaign) (pp. 228-251). Wiesbaden, Germany: VS-Verlag.

Kim, Sei-Hill, Scheufele, Dietram A., and Shanahan, James (2002). Think about it this way: Attribute agenda-setting and the publics evaluation of a local issue. Journalism and Mass Communication Quarterly 79 (1), 7-25.

Kinder, Donald R. (1998). Communication and opinion. Annual Review of Political Science 1, 167-197.

Kiousis, Spiro, Bantimaroudis, Philemon, and Hyun Ban (1999). Candidate image attributes: Experiments on the substantive dimension of second level agenda setting. Communication Research 26 (4), 414-428.

Krosnick, Jon A. & Kinder, Donald R. (1990). Altering the foundations of support for the president through priming. American Political Science Review 8 (2), 497-509.

Ku, Gyotae, Kaid, Lynda Lee, and Pfau (2004). The impact of Web site campaigning on traditional news media and public information Processing. Journalism & Mass Communication Quarterly 80 (3), 528-547.

Lopez-Escobar, Esteban, McCombs, Maxwell, and Lennon, Federico Rey (1998). Two levels of agenda setting among advertising and news in the 1995 Spanish elections. Political Communication 15, 225-238.

McCombs and Shaw (1972). The agenda setting function of mass media. Public Opinion Quarterly 36(2), 176-187.

McCombs, Maxwell and Shaw, Donald (1993). The evolution of agenda setting research: Twenty-five years in the marketplace. Journal of Communication 43, 58-67.

McCombs, Maxwell and Ghanem, Salma I. (2003). The convergence of agenda setting and framing. Reese, S.D., Gandy, O.H, Jr., & Grant, A.E. Framing Public Life: Perspectives on the Media and our Understandings
of the Social World. Mahwah, NJ: Lawrence Erlbaum Associates, pp. 67-81.

McCombs, Messaris, P., & Abraham, L. (2001). The Role of Images in Framing News Stories. In: Framing Public Life: Perspectives on Media and Our Understanding of the Social World. Reese, S. D., Gandy, H. H., & Gant, A. E. (Eds.) Mahwah, New Jersey: 215-226.

Miller, M. M., & Riechert, B. P. (2001). The Spiral of Opportunity and Frame Resonance: Mapping the Issue Cycle in News and Public Discourse. In: Framing Public Life: Perspectives on Media and Our Understanding of the Social World. Reese, S. D., Gandy, H. H., & Gant, A. E. (Eds.)
Mahwah, New Jersey: 107-121.

Maxwell, Lopez-Escobar, Esteban, and Llamas, Juan Pablo (2000). Setting the agenda of attributes in the 1996 Spanish general election. Journal of Communication, 77-92.

Mutz, Diana C. and Soss, Joe (1997). Reading public opinion: The influence of news coverage on perceptions of public sentiment. Public Opinion Quarterly 61, 431-451.

Noelle-Neumann, Elisabeth (1980). The public opinion research correspondent. Public Opinion Quarterly 44, 585-597.

Pan, Zhongdang and Kosicki, Gerald M. (1997). Priming and media impact on the evaluations of the president's performance. Communication Research 24 (1), pp. 3-30.

Pan, Z., & Kosicki, G. M. (2001). Framing as a Strategic Action in Public Deliberation. In: Framing Public Life: Perspectives on Media and Our Understanding of the   Social World. Reese, S. D., Gandy, H. H., & Gant, A. E. (Eds.) Mahwah, New Jersey: 35-64.

Reese, Stephen. D. (1991). Setting the media's agenda: A power balance perspective. In J. A. Anderson (Ed.), Communication Yearbook, 14, pp. 303-399. Newbury Park, CA: Sage Publications.

Reese, Stephen, Gandy, Oscar H, Jr., & Grant, August E. (2003). Framing Public Life: Perspectives on the Media and our Understandings of the Social World. Mahwah, NJ: Lawrence Erlbaum Associates. Version One: 15 January 2008.

Roberts, M. and McCombs, M. (1994). Agenda setting and political advertising: Origins of the news agenda. Political Communication 11, 249-262.

Roberts, M.S., & Williams A.P. (2003). Lockbox and Fuzzy Math: Associations of Viewers' Debate Recall and Voter Behavior in L.L. Kaid, J. C. Tedesco, D., Bystrom, and M.S. McKinney (Eds.) The Millennium Edition: Communication in the 2000 Campaigns (pp. 73-86). Lanham, MD: Rowman & Littlefield.

Robinson, Michael J. (1976). Public affairs television and the growth of political malaise: the case of "The selling of the Pentagon." *American Political Science Review* 70, 409-432

Rogers and Dearing (1993). The anatomy of agenda-setting research. Journal of Communication 43(2), 68-84.

Scheufele, D.A. (1999). Framing as a Theory of Media Effects. Journal of Communication Research, Winter 1999: 103-122.

Scheufele, Dietram A. (2000). Agenda-setting, priming, and framing revisited: Another look at cognitive effects of political communication. Mass Communication & Society 3 (2/3), 297-317.

Tankard, J. W. (2001). The Empirical Approach to the Study of Media Framing. In: Framing Public Life: Perspectives on Media and Our Understanding of the Social World. Reese, S. D., Gandy, H. H., & Gant, A. E. (Eds.) Mahwah, New Jersey: 107-121.

Tedesco, J. C. (2005). Intercandidate agenda setting in the 2004 Democratic presidential primary. American Behavioral Scientist, (49), 92-113.

Tedesco, John C. (2001). Issue and Strategy Agenda-Setting in the 2000 Presidential Primaries. American Behavioral Scientist, 44, (12), pp. 2048-2067.

Tipton, I., Haney, R.D. & Baseheart, J.R. (1975). Media agenda-setting in city and state election campaigns. Journalism Quarterly, 52, 15-22.

Turk, J. V., & Franklin, B. (1987). Information Subsidies: Agenda Setting Traditions. Public Relations Review, 13 (4), 29-41.

Weaver, David (1984). Media agenda-setting and public opinion: Is there a link? Bostrom, R.N. (ed.), Communication Yearbook 8, Beverly Hills, SA: Sage, p. 680-691.

Weaver, David, McCombs, Maxwell, and Shaw, Donald (2004). Agenda setting research: Issues, attributes, and influences. Lynda Lee Kaid (Ed.) Handbook of Political Communication Research. Mahwah, NJ: Lawrence
Erlbaum Associates, pp. 257-282.

Williams, A.P., & Maiorescu, R. (2015). Evaluating Candidate Campaign E-mail Messages in U.S. Presidential Election 2012. In Hendricks, John Allen & Schill, Dan (Eds.): Presidential Campaigning and Social Media.
New York: Oxford University Press.

Williams, A.P., & Serge, E. (2011). Evaluating Candidate Campaign E-mail Messages in U.S. Presidential Election 2008. In Hendricks, John Allen & Kaid, Lynda Lee (Eds.): Techno Politics in Presidential Campaigning. New Voices, New Technologies, and New Voters (pp. 44-57). New York: Routledge.

Williams, A.P., Kaid, L.L., Landreville, K.D., Fernandes, J., Yun, H.J., & Bagley, A., & Urriste, S. (2008). The Representation of the European Union Elections in News Media Coverage around the World. In L.L. Kaid, (Ed.) The Expansion Election: Communicating Shared Sovereignty in the 2004 European Parliamentary Elections (pp. 153-173). New York: Peter Lang Publishing.

Williams, A.P. (2006). Self-Referential and Opponent Based Framing: Candidate E-Mail Strategies in Election 2004. In A.P. Williams, & J.C. Tedesco, (Eds.) The Internet Election: Perspectives on the Web's Role in Campaign 2004 (pp. 83-98). Lanham, MD: Rowman & Littlefield Publishers.

Williams, A.P. (2006). Net Narcissism: Leading TV News Web sites' Self Reflexive Coverage during Operation Iraqi Freedom in R.D. Berenger (Ed.) Cybermedia Go to War—Role of Non-traditional Media in the 2003 Iraq War and its Aftermath (pp. 372-382). Spokane, WA: Marquette Books.

Williams, A.P., & Kaid, L.L. (2006). Media Framing of the European Parliamentary Elections: A View from the United States in M. Maier and J. Tenscher (Eds.) Campaigning in Europe—Campaigning for Europe: Political Parties, Campaigns, Mass Media and the European Parliament Elections 2004 (pp. 295-304). Berlin: LIT Publishers.

Williams, A.P. (2005). The Main Frame: Assessing the Role of the Internet in the 2004 U.S. Presidential Contest in R.E. Denton (Ed.) The 2004 Presidential Campaign: A Communication Perspective (pp.241-254). Lanham, MD: Rowman & Littlefield.

Williams, A.P., Martin, J.D., Trammell, K.D., Landreville, K., & Ellis, C. (2004). Late night talk shows and war: Entertaining and informing through humor in R.D. Berenger (Ed.) Global Media Go to War (pp. 131-138). Spokane, WA: Marquette Books.

Williams, A.P., & Kaid, L.L. (2006). Media Framing of the European Parliamentary Elections: A View from the United States in M. Maier and Tenscher, J. (Eds.) Campaigning in Europe— Campaigning for Europe: Political Parties, Campaigns, Mass Media and the European Parliament Elections 2004 (pp. 295-304). Berlin: LIT Publishers.

Willnat, Lars (2000). Agenda setting and priming: Conceptual links and differences. Donald Shaw, Maxwell McCombs, and David H. Weaver (eds.) Communication and Democracy, London: Lawrence Erlbaum Associates, pp. 51-66.

Chapter Three: Yoga

Light on Yoga by B.K.S. Iyengar:
https://www.amazon.com/s/?ie=UTF8&keywords=light+on+Yog
a&tag=googhydr-
20&index=aps&hvadid=241929004945&hvpos=1t1&hvnetw=g&
hvrand=6128420301345132197&hvpone=&hvptwo=&hvqmt=e
&hvdev=c&hvdvcmdl=&hvlocint=&hvlocphy=9011012&hvtargi
d=kwd-300060232243&ref=pd_sl_6vugs9r9v2_e_p37

The Yoga Sutras of Patanjali [Sri Swami Satchidananda]:
https://books.google.com/books/about/The_Yoga_Sutras_of_Pat
anjali.html?id=NrhDAAAAYAAJ&printsec=frontcover&source
=kp_read_button#v=onepage&q&f=false

Yoga Den: https://www.Yoga-den.com/

Yoga Journal: "Yoga Poses & Asanas - Basic to Advanced:"
https://www.Yogajournal.com/poses

"Pranayama (Breathing) Exercises & Poses"
https://www.Yogajournal.com/poses/types/pranayama

Andrew's Personal Practice

This basic structure can be made gentler by removing some of the more active shapes and movements or can be made more rigorous by adding to it and speeding up your pace. Find what works best for you. There are many resources online, and I am teaching classes regularly via zoom for Yoga Den Fleming Island. You can register online or using their app: https://yoga-den.com/fleming-island-schedule/

Center seated (Lotus Pose), set an intention, and go to your breath. Use this time to think about your relationship with yourself, others, and the world around you.
https://www.yogajournal.com/poses/lotus-pose

Gentle Neck Movements

Shoulder Shrugs and Rolls

Full Body Stretch on your Back

Hug Knees to Chest and Massage Back

Warm Ankles, Knees, and Hips

Roll Up to Seated

Seated Spinal Twist

Side Stretches

Table (*Bharmanasana*) http://www.yogabasics.com/asana/table-pose/

Cat (*Marjyasana*) and Cow (*Bitilasana*) Stretches
https://yogadigest.com/the-synchronization-of-breath-movement-catcow/

Thread The Needle (*Parsva Balasana*)
https://www.gaia.com/article/thread-needle-pose-parsva-balasana

Spinal Balance (dandayamna bharmanasana)
http://www.yogabasics.com/asana/balancing-table/

Puppy Stretch (*Uttana Shishosana*)
https://www.yogajournal.com/poses/extended-puppy-pose

Downward Dog (*Adho Mukha Svanasana)*
https://www.yogaoutlet.com/guides/how-to-do-downward-facing-dog-in-yoga

Forward Fold (*Uttanasana*)
https://www.yogajournal.com/poses/standing-forward-bend

Gentle Standing Back Bend (*Anuvittasana*)
http://www.yogabasics.com/asana/standing-backbend/

Mountain (*Tadasana*)
https://www.verywellfit.com/mountain-pose-tadasana-3567127

Crescent of Half Moon (*Urdhva Hastasana*)
http://www.yogabasics.com/asana/crescent-moon/

Tree (*Vrksasana)*
https://www.drweil.com/health-wellness/balanced-living/exercise-fitness/tree-pose/

Sun Salutation A (*Surya Namaskara A*)
https://www.yogaoutlet.com/guides/how-to-do-sun-salutation-a-in-yoga

Chair (*Utkatasana*)   https://www.yogajournal.com/poses/chair-pose

Chair Twist/ Revolved Chair Pose (*Parivrtta Utkatasana*)
https://www.yogajournal.com/practice/5-steps-strong-alignment-revolved-chair-pose

Sun Salutation B (*Surya Namaskara)*
https://www.yogaoutlet.com/guides/how-to-do-sun-salutation-b-in-yoga

Warrior I (*Virabhadrasana I*)
http://www.yogabasics.com/asana/warrior-i/

Warrior II (*Virabhadrasana II*)
http://www.yogabasics.com/asana/warrior-ii/

Extended Side Angle (*Parsvakonasana)*
https://www.yogaoutlet.com/guides/how-to-do-extended-side-angle-pose-in-yoga

Triangle (*Trikonasana)*
https://www.ekhartyoga.com/more-yoga/yoga-poses/extended-triangle-pose#

Pyramid (*Parsvottanasana)*
https://www.yogajournal.com/poses/intense-side-stretch-pose

Warrior III (*Virabhadrasana III*)
http://www.yogabasics.com/asana/warrior-iii/

Three Point Balance

Half Moon (*Adha Chandrasana*)
https://www.ekhartyoga.com/articles/5-tips-for-half-moon-pose

Revolved Half Moon (*Parivrtta Ardha Chandrasana)*
https://yogainternational.com/article/view/revolved-half-moon

Wild Thing (*Camatkarasana*) Feel free to flip your dog!
https://www.yogajournal.com/poses/wild-thing

Plank
https://www.yogajournal.com/poses/plank-pose

Side Plank (*Vasisthasana*)
https://www.yogajournal.com/poses/side-plank-pose

Thread the Needle in Side Plank

Cobra (*Bhujangasana*)
https://www.yogajournal.com/practice/cobra-pose

Child's Pose (*Balasana)*
https://www.yogaoutlet.com/guides/how-to-do-child_s-pose-in-yoga

Pigeon (*Eka Pada Rajakapotasana*)
https://www.verywellfit.com/pigeon-pose-eka-pada-rajakapotasana-3567103

Bound Angle (*Baddha Konasana*)
http://www.yogabasics.com/asana/bound-angle/

Full or Double Pigeon (*Agnistambhasana*)
https://www.gaia.com/article/double-pigeon-or-fire-log-pose-agnistambhasana

Staff Pose (*Dandasana*)
https://www.yogauonline.com/yoga-pose-primer/building-core-strength-dandasana-staff-pose

Seated Spinal Twist or Half Lord of the Fishes Pose (*Matsyendrasana*)
https://www.yogajournal.com/poses/half-lord-of-the-fishes-pose

Head-to-Knee Forward Fold (*Janu Sirsasana*)
https://www.yogajournal.com/practice/4-steps-to-master-janu-sirsasana

Forward Seated Fold/Posterior Stretch (*Paschimottanasana*)
https://www.yogajournal.com/poses/seated-forward-bend

Upward Facing Boat (*Navasana*)
https://www.yogaoutlet.com/guides/how-to-do-boat-pose-in-yoga

Bridge (*Setu Bandha Sarvangasana*)
https://www.yogajournal.com/poses/perfect-your-bridge-pose-in-6-steps

Knees-to-Chest Post (*Apanasana) Give Yourself a Hug!*
https://www.yogaoutlet.com/guides/how-to-do-knees-to-chest-pose-in-yoga

Half Shoulder Stand (*Ardha Sarvangasana*) or other Inversion, as restorative or advanced as you enjoy
http://www.yogabasics.com/asana/half-shoulder-stand/

Happy Baby (*Ananda Balasana*)
https://www.gaia.com/article/happy-baby-pose-ananda-balasana

Alternate Knees to Chest (*Apanasana*)
http://www.feelgoodyogavictoria.com/learning-centre/yoga/knee-chest-apanasana-pose/

Supine Spinal Twist (*Supta Matsyendrasana*) ending in Supine Tree in each eirection
https://www.yogaoutlet.com/guides/how-to-do-reclined-spinal-twist-in-yoga

Yoga Nidra relaxation of your whole body from your toes to your head.

Chakra's Meditation

White Light Healing Meditation

Corpse Pose (*Savasana*)
https://www.yogajournal.com/practice/corpse-pose

Yoga Alliance: https://www.Yogaalliance.org/

Carol DeVault Lahey guided my research about training the mind to file things away and intentional denial of negative stimuli.

Heather Fisse guided my research about Yoga and evaluating energy and outcomes.

Heather Fisse and Jon Repole taught me about Ayuveda and the Doshas in my advanced teacher training at Yoga Den which has helped guide my choices in terms of Yoga Practice.

Acknowledgments

There are many people who helped me during this process and my growth as a Yoga instructor. Below are people who directly helped me with the concepts for this book.

It has taken me about four years to finish this short book, and the original idea that sparked my interest in this concept was first introduced to me on Thanksgiving morning by Alyson Foreacre at a Turkey Day Detox practice sponsored by Yoga Den. This book directly grew out of the final paper I wrote for my 300-hour advanced teacher training at Yoga Den. Alyson and her husband, Chip, have been incredible mentors and friends to me and have made it possible for me to launch a new career and improve myself a great deal. I am very grateful

The 200-hour and 300-hour teacher training I received at Yoga Den is on par with any training I've received during my academic and professional work at Colleges, Universities and Foundations in the United States and Europe. The training from Yoga Den helped me advance my work with Framing theory that began under the direction of Dr. Lynda Lee Kaid at the University of Florida, College of Journalism and Communications and continued through my work as a professor in the Department of Communication at Virgina Tech. Applying Framing Theory to my study and teaching of yoga helped me personally and has resonated with my students and clients.

Khristi Keefe-Bowens who gave me the opportunity to be a part of Much Ado about Books and Yoga 2018 – a wonderful friend and colleague.

Heather Fisse – who encouraged me to weave these concepts from my writing more directly into my teaching and view the process more holistically. Heather is great friend, Yoga teacher, and Coach who helped guide me through this process.

Dr. Carol Devault Lahey– a skilled Psychologist who helped me recover from trauma, guided me through a life transition, and became a role model and friend.

Mary Chase – a great friend and my first Yoga teacher who helped me start this journey.

Debi Boyette - my sweet friend who motivated me with this Yoga journey right from the start and designed the Williams Press logo.

Hila Head - who encouraged me to start Yoga when I first moved back from Virginia and has been an incredible support and close friend to me. She also came to my first Yoga class at Yoga Den Avondale.

Mary Daley – a great friend who has helped me much personally and professionally and listened to me brainstorm this and other projects many times. Mary also came to take my first Yoga class.

Jon Repole help with setting intentions, discissing the work of Joseph Campbell, and encouragment with this project.

My Brother, Grady H. Williams, Jr., LL.M. has helped me immensely by providing me much freedom and flexibility to pursue my training, teaching opportunities, and working with clients while I also work for his Law Firm as its Public Relations and Social Media Manager. This continuation of my PR career has given me many opportunities to use and grow my skills and to apply and share the concepts in this book.

While working on this book, I had the opportunity to present about Mindfulness and Yoga at the Shepard Center with our firm's Associate Attorney, Alison E. Hickman. This presentation to a group of seniors who were very interested in, and practiced Mindfulness Meditation and Yoga, helped me get valuable feedback and see how useful these practices and Framing are for people of all ages. Alison has helped me with my writing and been a great source of encouragement.

Paula Emery, a good friend a colleague who I've enjoyed working with on Marketing and Public Relations. She's been an ongoing motivator and positive supporter of my endeavors.

Joan Tymick – editor, friend, Yoga student who helped me so much with this project.

Liz Robbins – friend, colleague, Yoga student who encouraged and motivated me with this book and as a Yoga instructor.

Chris Dew -- a friend who I went to UNF with while we were working on our Master's Degrees in English Literature who helped to edit this book and encourage me efforts in combining of these three disciplines.

Andrea and Christopher Hernandez – owners of Yoga Den Fleming Island who have become friends and encouragers.

Jen Williams – former owner of Yoga Den World Golf Village – who has become a friend and made much possible for me.

Beth Mihaly – friend, inspiration, Yoga student, and co-author of *The Book of Empowerment*—a book that grew out of this project and our awesome Yoga sessions together.

Jurgen Maier – a friend and college who I conducted research with regarding the effects of what order a group of photos had on viewers in terms of frame tone. This study helped me advance my interests in the content and effects of visual Framing.

Frank Esser and Paul D'Angelo – whose seminal work on meta-communication guided my dissertation at UF and work still informs my understanding of framing.

To all my friends, teachers, students, and colleagues. Thank you, all.

Made in the USA
Middletown, DE
05 January 2023

21111350R00056